YOGA OF PERFECT SIGHT

WITH
LETTERS OF SRI AUROBINDO

Dr. R. S. AGARWAL

SRI AUROBINDO ASHRAM
PONDICHERRY

First edition 1971
Second edition (Revised and Enlarged) 1974
Third edition (Facsimile) 1977
Tenth impression 2005

Price: Rs 55
ISBN 81-7058-209-1

Published by Sri Aurobindo Ashram Publication Department,
Pondicherry - 605 002
Website: http://sabda.sriaurobindoashram.org

Printed at Sri Aurobindo Ashram Press, Pondicherry
PRINTED IN INDIA

EDITOR'S NOTE

This book is a collection of articles written by my father, Dr. R. S. Agarwal. Most of the articles were first published in *Mother India*, a monthly journal of Sri Aurobindo Ashram, Pondicherry. The last chapter includes letters of Sri Aurobindo about eyesight and Yogic vision.

The author has added some more experiences in this new edition.

DR. J. AGARWAL M.B., B.S., D.O.M.S.

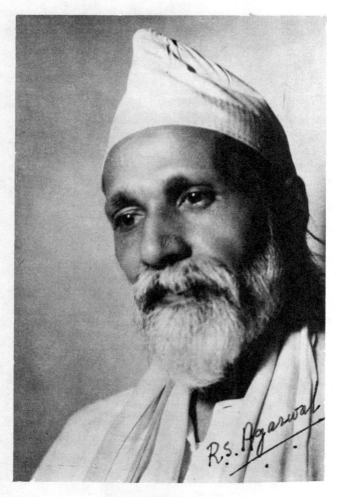

Dr. R. S. AGARWAL
THE DISCOVERER OF A SYNTHESIS IN
OPHTHALMIC SCIENCE

CONTENTS

CHAPTER I

INTRODUCTORY

Almost every eye specialist of the world believes that for refractive errors there is not only no cure but practically no preventive also. From such a belief any rational mind will conclude that science is in a very imperfect stage. What some writers on Ophthalmology wrote two hundred years back about the incurability of the refractive ailments, is continuing as a dogma even today, in the days of advanced science. We are so much hypnotised by the assertions of the old authorities that we do not care to make any experiment or do some research on the subject. And if anyone comes forward to say that cases of errors of refraction can be improved without glasses, we begin to doubt and without any study discard his explanation. Such is the condition of our mind which is supposed to be scientific. A scientific mind is always open to admit a truth or a fact.

The old writers tell us that the visual organ of man was never intended for the uses to which it is put now. In the early ages there was no school, no printing press, no electric light and no moving pictures. In those days the eye served the needs of the human animal perfectly. Man was a hunter, a farmer, a fighter; he needed only distant vision for which no muscular action was required. It is in near vision that some muscular action is required to correct the focusing, but at that time the use of eyes for near was rare and of very short duration.

When man learned how to communicate his thoughts to others by means of written and printed forms, there came some undeniably new demands upon the eye, affecting at first only a few people but gradually including more and more, and now in the most advanced countries the great mass of the population suffers from defective vision. Since the tallow candle has been displaced by the various forms of artificial lighting and the moving pictures have come in to use, almost every one suffers from some form of refractive error.

The prevailing method of treatment for the errors of refraction is by means of compensating lenses. But very little has ever been claimed except that these contrivances neutralise the effects of the various conditions for which they are prescribed as a crutch enables a lame man to walk. In the case of myopia Dr. Sidler Huguenin expresses the opinion that glasses and all methods at our command are "of but little avail" in peventing either the progress of the error of refraction or the development of the very serious complications with which it is often associated.

This incurability of errors of refraction is based on the theory that the eye changes its focus for vision at different distances by altering the curvature of the lens. And both myopia and hypermetropia are supposed to be permanent conditions.

While examining thirty thousand pairs of eyes, Dr. W.H. Bates, the pioneer Ophthalmologist of New York, observed many cases of defective vision who recovered spontaneously, or changed their form of ailment. Dr. Bates was unable either to ignore these facts, or to satisfy himself with the orthodox explanations. It seemed to him that if a statement is a truth it must always be a truth. If errors of refraction are incurable they should never recover or change their form spontaneously. In seeking for light Dr. Bates undertook a series of observations upon the eyes of human beings and lower animals, the results of which convinced him that the lens is not a factor in accommodation. The eye adjusts its focus for different distances just like a camera, by a change in the length of the organ, and this alteration is brought about by the action of the external eye muscles called oblique muscles. We mention here some very important discoveries by Dr. Bates regarding the refractive error. The modern ophthalmologists should study these discoveries and if necessary repeat Dr. Bates experiments as his work needs further investigation.

Discoveries of Dr. Bates

1. Myopia and hypermetropia could be produced at will.
2. Myopia was not caused by reading but by a strain to see distant objects.
3. Strain at the near point caused hypermetropia.
4. No error of refraction was ever a constant condition.
5. Lower degrees of errors of refraction were curable while higher degrees could be improved.
6. Reading fine print when it can be done without any discomfort proves extremely beneficial.
7. Preservation of good eyesight is almost impossible without eye education and mental relaxation.

The most remarkable discovery of Dr. Bates is:

FINE PRINT IS A BENEFIT TO THE EYES WHILE LARGE PRINT IS A MENACE. The reason is that while reading fine print one sees a tiny area at a time, while in reading large print one has to see a large area at a time and the eye feels strain in such an attempt. Reading of fine print when it can be done without discomfort, has invariably proved to be beneficial — and all the more if good light and candle light are used alternately.

Often it is surprising how quickly the vision begins to improve by Dr. Bates, simple methods of eye education. For example, a girl student of Sri Aurobindo International Centre of Education, whose eyesight had failed both for far and near, recovered normal eyesight in about a week's time. And a teacher at the Centre, whose left eye had been blind since childhood, regained normal sight within two months with regular eye exercises for about two hours a day. Almost all semiblind patients respond well to this treatment and they can be saved from total blindness.

Cases of high myopia, detachment of retina, macular degeneration, optic atrophy, retinitis, early glaucoma, early cataract, amblyopia, squint, retinitis pigmentosa etc., have derived great benefit by the system of eye education and mental relaxation. Most of the cases suffering from severe headache are quickly relieved by resting the eyes and mind through relaxation exercises. Inflammation of the eyes get much relief by sun treatment.

Strange as it may seem, Dr. Bates system of eye education is almost dead in the land of its origin — America — but it lives and grows in India. Dr. Agarwal's Eye Institutes in Delhi and Madras, and the School For Perfect Eyesight at Pondicherry are working on Dr. Bates lines.

We believe that all the systems of medicine and methods of treatment have their utility. Hence for practical working we have developed a synthesis so as to give most benefit to the eye patients. Such a synthesis has been explained in *Mind and Vision* and *Secrets of Indian Medicine*.

As there has been a considerable demand for a practical book on eye education and perfect eyesight, an attempt has been made to present the subject in a simple and interesting way.

Definitions

NORMAL VISION: is perfect sight at all distances. The Snellen test card is the standard for testing the vision. When the twenty feet line of the card can be read at twenty feet or further, and fine print can be read at six inches or less, one has normal vision.

MYOPIA OR NEAR-SIGHTEDNESS: The vision for near objects is good, while the distant vision is impaired.

HYPERMETROPIA OR FAR-SIGHTEDNESS: The sight is not so good at a near point as it is for more distant objects.

PRESBYOPIA OR OLD AGE SIGHT: The vision is imperfect when the patient tries to read fine print at a near point. The distant vision may or may not be good.

ASTIGMATISM: is an imperfect curvature of the eye. Usually the front part of the eye has a curve which is different from all the other curves.

CATARACT: is an opacity of the lens in the pupils, which interferes with good vision.

MEMORY, OR IMAGINATION, is the ability to see or recall letters or other objects, when the eyes are closed or open.

THE SNELLEN TEST CARD: has letters printed in varying sizes. The smallest letter on the card is a measure of the vision.

FINE PRINT: is one of the smallest types used in printing and helps to improve the vision if it is read every day.

BLINKING: is a short and gentle movement of the eyelids.

Fundamentals

By W. H. Bates, M. D.

1. Central Fixation is seeing best where you are looking.

2. Favourable conditions: Light may be bright or dim. The distance of the print from the eyes, where seen best, also varies with people.

3. Shifting: With normal sight the eyes are moving all the time.

4. Swinging: When the eyes move slowly or rapidly from side to side, stationary objects appear to move in the opposite direction.

5. Long Swing: Stand with the feet about one foot apart, turn the body to the right—at the same time lifting the heel of the left foot. Do not move the head or eyes or pay any attention to the apparent movement of stationary objects. Now place the left heel on the floor, turn the body to the left, raising the heel of the right foot. Alternate.

6. Drifting Swing: When practising this swing, one pays no attention to the clearness of stationary objects, which appear to be moving. The eyes wander from point to point slowly, easily, or lazily, so that the stare or strain may be avoided.

7. Variable Swing: Hold the forefinger of one hand six inches from the right eye and about the same distance to the right, look straight ahead and move the head a short distance from side to side. The finger appears to move.

8. Stationary Objects Moving: By moving the head and eyes a short distance from side to side, being sure to blink, one can imagine stationary objects to be moving.

9. Memory: Improving the memory of letters and other objects improves the vision for everything.

10. Imagination: We see only what we think we see, or what we imagine. We can only imagine what we remember.

11. Rest: All cases of imperfect sight are improved by closing the eyes and resting them.

12. Palming: The closed eyes may be covered with the palm of one or both hands.

13. Blinking: The normal eye blinks or closes and opens very frequently.

14. Mental Pictures: As long as one is awake one has all kinds of memories of mental pictures. If these pictures are remembered easily, perfectly, the vision is benefited.

Suggestions

1. If the vision of the patient is improved under the care of the doctor and the patient, when he leaves the clinic, neglects to practise what he is told to do at home, the treatment has been of no benefit whatever. The improved vision was only temporary. Faithful practice permanently improves the vision.

2. If the patient conscientiously practises the methods, as advised by the doctor, his vision always improves.

3. When a patient suffers with cataract, palming is usually the best method of treatment, and should be practised many times every day.

4. All patients with imperfect sight unconsciously stare, and should be reminded by those who are near them to blink often. To stare is a strain. Strain is the cause of imperfect sight.

5. While sitting, do not look up without raising your chin. Always turn your head in the direction in which you look.

6. Do not make an effort to see things more clearly. If you let your eyes alone, things will clear up by themselves.

7. Do not look at anything longer than a fraction of a second without shifting.

8. While reading shift your head and eyes together from side to side with gentle blinking.

9. When you are conscious of your eyes while looking at objects at any time, it causes discomfort and lessens your vision.

10. It is very important that you learn how to imagine stationary objects to be moving, as you seem to observe while moving in a train.

11. Palming is a help, and I suggest that you palm for a few minutes several times a day. To palm at bed-time induces good sleep.

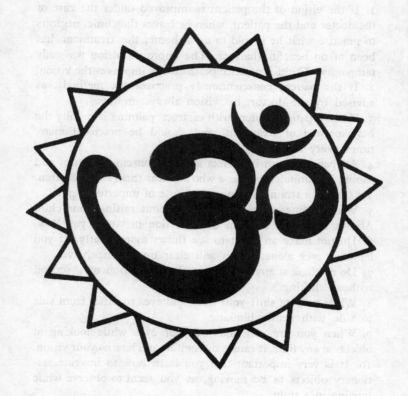

OM CHART

Central Fixation on Om Chart

When the normal eye sees a thing, it sees only that part of the thing best on which it fixes itself and the other parts are not seen so well.

Shift the sight on the angular lines of Om chart. Note that each line regarded appears best. While shifting the sight from one line to another, move the head and sight together. Blink at each corner.

Sun treatment and Dark Glasses

Most ophthalmologists prescribe dark glasses to all those who suffer from the brightness of light and feel the glare while walking about. This practice, in my opinion has been overdone. A patient was practically blind in bright sunlight. He went to a great many eye clinics and eye doctors and all they did for him was to give stronger dark glasses. In time these dark glasses did not give him any relief. Instead of being helpful to his weak eyes, the glasses had the effect of making them more sensitive to the light than they had ever been before. It has been my experience that almost all persons who wear dark glasses sooner or later develop some eye trouble. The human eye needs the light in order to maintain its efficiency. The use of eye-shades and protections of all kinds from the light is injurious to the eyes. For natural protection the eyelids are there on the eyes. When the person keeps the lids moving and does proper blinking the eyes do not feel any glare in bright light.

Sunlight is as necessary to normal eye as are rest and relaxation. If it is possible, start the day by exposing the eyes to the sun — just a few minutes at a time will help. Get accustomed to the strong light of the sun by letting it shine on your closed eyelids. It is good to move the head slightly from side to side while taking sun treatment, in order to prevent straining. One should not take too much sun treatment as the heat of the sun will cause discomfort.

The Eye and the Camera

The eye is an animate miniature photographic camera. It has a lens, iris (diaphragm) and a retina or film for receiving the images. The normal eye never makes an effort to see.

The eye adjusts its focus from far to near just like the camera by lengthening itself through the action of the oblique muscles. This adjustment of the focus is called accommodation. So we can say that in accommodation the eye-ball is lengthened. The lens has nothing to do with accommodation, it does not change its surface. It is only by an effort can one prevent the eye from elongating at the near-point.

When the eye looks at 20 ft. or beyond without any effort or strain, no adjustment is necessary; then it is said that the eye is at rest. The shape of the eye-ball cannot be altered during distant vision without strain.

But there is one great difference between the eye and the camera, and that difference is in the film. The film of the camera is equally sensitive in all its parts, but the retina of the eye has a point of maximum sensitiveness, which is called Central Spot or macula lutea. Due to this increased sensitiveness the eye sees best where it looks at, and this quality of the eye is called Central fixation.

The retina has a layer of rods and cones. The cones work in light, while the rods work in darkness. A cock's eye has only cones, a bat's eye has only rods, but in the higher animals or in man both rods and cones are present. The macula lutea is full of cones, there is no rod. The extreme end of the retina has only rods, there are no cones. In between both rods and cones are present.

The eye is a sensory organ and functions without effort like other sensory organs; as you hear or smell, so you see. When there is no effort to see, the function of the eye is normal and the eye has perfect eyesight, the image is focused correctly on the retina. But the moment the normal eye makes an effort to see, it ceases to be normal. So, there may be myopia, hypermetropia with or without astigmatism.

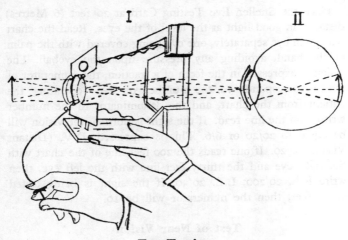

Eye Testing

When a person presents himself for treatment, a record of his name, age and address is to be made. Then one hears the history and complaints of the patient and, if necessary puts him a few cross-questions. The next procedure is to test the distant vision on the Snellen Test Card without and with glasses. Then the near sight is tested on the reading test type without and with glasses. Such records of eyesight are to be made from time to time during the course of the treatment. They give the information of the improvement achieved. In some cases the improvement is so unconscious that the patient feels no improvement unless the records of vision are compared before him.

Test of Distant Vision

Place the Snellen Eye Testing Card at 20 feet (6 Metres) distance in good light at the level of the eyes. Read the chart with each eye separately, one eye being covered with the palm of the hand, avoiding any pressure upon the eyeball. The vision is expressed in the form of a fraction, the numerator of which corresponds to the number of feet separating the patient from the chart, and the denominator to the number written on the line read. If the sight is normal, the vision will be equal to 20/20 or 6/6. This is expressed: D.V. (Distant Vision) 20/20. If one reads the 200 feet line of the chart with the right eye and the thirty feet line with the left eye, then write R.E. 20/200; L.E. 20/30. If the sight is being tested at 10 feet, then the numerator will be 10.

Test of Near Vision

Test the sight on the Fundamental Reading Test Type. Hold the test card at 9 inches. Read it with each eye, covering the other with the palm of the hand. The vision is expressed by F (Fundamentals) followed by the number corresponding to the smallest type which one can read. Suppose one reads No. 4 of the Fundamentals at 9 inches with the right eye, then write, R.E. F4 at 9 inches.

Care of Eyes: A Dialogue

Sarla is an intelligent girl. Her eyes are beautiful. She is fond of music and knows the art of sewing. She is on a visit to the Sri Aurobindo Ashram and enjoys the peaceful atmosphere. Her brother Ramesh is a young man of 25, his marriage is near. Sarla wants to stitch a suit for her brother. She has bought a piece of silk from the Auro Silk House.

Every morning after her prayers in the Sri Aurobindo Mandir she sits in the verandah to stitch the suit. After a few days she begins to feel a strain in her eyes and a pain in her head. One day she has intense headache and the pain in her eyes is so bad that she puts herself to bed. Her mother enters.

Mother —   My darling, my darling,
                    How are you?
                    My little one, my little one,
                    what pains you?

Sarla —   Ma, pain in the head,
                    Pain in the eyes
                    Has put me to bed,
                    Forbids me to rise.

The mother directs Sarla to go to an eye doctor. The doctor examines Sarla's eyes carefully but finds nothing wrong, yet he has prescribed glasses of plus 0.5.

Sarla now stitches the cloth with her glasses on but after a few days the headache and pain increase, her mother is greatly worried, she requests her husband to take Sarla to Dr. Agarwal.

Seth Ratanji is Sarla's father. He has arranged an appointment with the doctor and brings the daughter to his eye clinic. The nurse receives them. The doctor writes down her name and age and address and her complaint of pain and headache. Sarla sits on the eye testing chair facing the eye chart which is at 20 feet distance from her eyes.

Doctor — Read that chart with the right eye.

Sarla (*Closing the left eye with the fingers*) — Very well.

Doctor — Not this way, cover the eye with the palm without any pressure on the eyeball.

Sarla (*now covering left eye with the palm*) — Yes, I can read up to 2 Q C O G D E C quite clearly.

Doctor (*writing 20/20,*) — Your right eye is normal. Now read with the left eye.

Sarla — Yes, 2 Q C line is quite clear.

The doctor then examines her eyes in the dark room and finds no defect. He and Sarla are now in the palming room. He puts her some questions.

Doctor — Can you tell me, Sarla, how you get strain and pain in your eyes?

Sarla — For some days I was stitching a cloth; it is at that time that the strain developed.

Doctor — Can you do stitching in my presence? Here are the needle and thread.

Sarla (*after a little stitching*) — Doctor, my eyes and head have become heavy.

Doctor — Leave it. I understand your trouble. Now make yourself relaxed. Close your eyes and cover them with the palms of your hands. Look, how I do it.

Sarla (*smiling*) — This is palming.

Doctor — How do you know?

Sarla — Our teacher, Mr. Joshi, told us in the class to do palming for a few minutes every day. His eyes have been greatly benefited by palming.

Doctor — Look at the blackness of the top letter of this chart or at the piece of black velvet placed on your pillow and then remember the black colour while palming. You will then observe that it is all perfectly dark before your eyes.

Sarla — Yes, I see it is all perfectly dark before my eyes.

Doctor — Continue palming for five minutes or till you feel quite relaxed.

Sarla (after palming) — Doctor, please, make me all right soon, I have to stitch a suit for my brother.

Doctor — You will find yourself quite all right tomorrow.

Sarla — Can you tell me, doctor, what is wrong with my eyes?

Doctor — Nothing wrong with your eyes except this that somehow you have developed a wrong habit of sewing. You don't blink, you don't move your sight with the movement of the needle. Just see, I am showing you the right method of sewing.

Sarla — This is very easy, I can also do sewing like that. (Sarla now does sewing in the right way, her sight moves with the movements of the needle.)

Doctor — One thing very important I'll tell you.

Sarla — What?

Doctor — Fine stitching and fine print reading are very beneficial to the eyes.

Sarla — But, doctor, a teacher of ours tells us that fine print reading is harmful.

Doctor — What is the age of this teacher?

Sarla — About 40 years.

Doctor — Usually at this age one feels a strain in reading fine print. That is why your teacher says so. But if one can make it a habit to read the same fine print daily, fine print reading will prove extremely beneficial.

Sarla — Is there any book of fine print?

Doctor — Here is fine print; can you read it?

Sarla — I can read it very well. Now please tell me something practical for the good of the school children.

Doctor — What is this in my hand?

Sarla — Eye Testing Chart.

Doctor — Put the eye chart on the wall of each class room and let the children read it silently from their seats with both eyes and with each eye separately, covering the other with the palm of the hand. Children should also be educated to do palming. This is enough to keep their eyes all right.

Sarla — This is quite pratical, it will need hardly 5 minutes. I will tell this fact to Mr. Joshi.

Doctor — Those who have bad eyesight may read it four or five times a day after palming.

Sarla — You said something about blinking. What is blinking?

Doctor — The upper lid makes a short and gentle movement; look at my eyes, see how I blink.

Sarla — I understand. Look at my blinking.

Doctor — This is winking, not blinking. Again see how I blink.

Sarla's father is greatly impressed by the doctor's knowledge and kind talk. He puts a big note in an envelope and presents it to the doctor along with the invitation to his son's marriage. Both Sarla and Seth Ratanji express their gratitude to the doctor and take leave.

Doctor Agarwal opens the envelope and finds a three figure

note in it. He feels very happy and sends this hundred rupee note to the Divine Mother for Ashram expenses. He knows that it is the Divine Grace that does miracles for his patients and that he is simply an instrument to give benefit to suffering humanity.

It is a fact that most of the eye troubles and other discomforts of the head are due to wrong use of the eyes and lack of relaxation. Mental relaxation is the key of success in life. If the students are taught how to read and write, how to see the cinema and do sewing, how to palm and read the chart, they will be free from mental strain and eye troubles, and show better progress all round.

ART OF SEEING

The School for Perfect Eyesight has developed a new technique called the 'art of seeing' for the cure of visual defects. Two Oriya girls, 10-years old, studying in Sri Aurobindo International Centre of Education, Pondicherry, had developed a condition of semi-blindness (Amblyopia). Their vision was found defective both for distance and near without any apparent cause and the glasses did not help them to see better. The teacher told us that the defective condition had developed after joining the school class. It is important to note that when children begin to learn unfamiliar things, letters or a language, they usually suffer from little or more of eye strain and mental strain due to the unfamiliarity of the lines and figures and letters. It is at this stage that visual defects usually start. And if children can be taught a few simple methods of eye education as blinking and palming etc., their defects will soon fade away and they will be blessed with perfect eyesight. Let me tell you how these two semiblind girls were cured in fifteen minutes by the art of seeing "view-cards and pictures."

I taught these girls the art of seeing pictures with the mind completely relaxed. I gave a view-card depicting a colourful picture of Taj Mahal to them. Soon the flatness began to disappear and the three-dimensional character of the picture was clearly perceived by the girls. With the mind relaxed, the picture appeared so beautiful to the eyes that their minds got deeply absorbed in seeing the Taj. They exclaimed, Lovely! Beautiful! the details of the picture were appearing sharply, they were observing their vision getting improved. Then when they were asked to read the Snellen Eye Testing Chart from 10ft and 20ft, they could easily read the normal line after a few attempts. They could also read the fine print which was impossible before. Since then they are maintaining permanent improvement. Formerly defective vision of this nature in children was cured in about two weeks but now by the art of seeing it was corrected in 15 minutes. Further experiments have proved that this exercise of mind and eyes proves very helpful in the improvement of eyesight in almost all cases who can successfully do it.

CHAPTER II

EYE STRAIN AND EYE EDUCATION

1. First understand how to see with an effort and without effort. It is a subtle point. Let the image come by itself to the eye, don't try to see. This is effortless seeing. The habit of making an effort to see is called eye strain. The normal eye ceases to be normal as soon as it makes an effort to see.

2. How to make an effort:

   a. Look intently or fix your gaze at a letter on the Snellen Eye Chart at 20 ft. distance.

   b. Try to read the letters of the chart at 20 ft. when it is placed in a dim light.

   c. Fix your gaze on a letter or a word at 10 inches.

   d. Try to read when the book is placed in dim light.

3. The strain to see at a distance causes lengthening of the eye-ball or myopia. Therefore, an effort to see at a distance will cause short sightedness or we can say like this:

   a. The normal eye will become myopic.

   b. The hypermetropic eye will become less hypermetropic or normal.

   c. Myopic eye will become more myopic.

4. The strain to see at a near point causes shortening or flattening of the eye-ball or hypermetropia. Therefore an effort to see at a near point will cause hypermetropia or we can say like this:

   a. The normal eye will become hypermetropic.

   b. The hypermetropic eye will become more hypermetropic.

   c. The myopic eye will become less myopic or normal.

5. When there is an effort to see or when one strains, the

eye does not blink in a normal way, usual blinking stops, or blinking turns into winking. Central fixation is disturbed, the capacity to see best is lessened. The look of the patient's eye is changed; it usually indicates strain.

6. Seeing unfamiliar objects, such as a map, unknown handwriting or script, always causes strain.

Eye Troubles

Function of the Eye: — The eye is one of the sense organs and the act of seeing is passive. Things are seen just as they are felt, or heard, or tasted, without effort or volition on the part of the subject. What we see through the eyes is simply the mind's interpretation of the retinal image.

Seeing is a complex process depending on five factors — object of seeing, organ of sight, sense function, interpretation of mind and attention of mind. The eye without the mind will mechanically photograph the image but will not interpret it. The mind without the eye can imagine the images previously seen, but will not tell you what you are seeing. Correct seeing must be a perfectly co-ordinated action between mind and eye.

Cause of Defective Eyesight: — The cause of defective eyesight is staring or making an effort to see. By an effort to see, the natural function of the eye is disturbed. If the eye stares at a distant object myopia is produced; and if the eye stares at a near point, hypermetropia is produced. It is a false belief that reading fine print causes myopia; in fact myopia is benefited by reading fine print. The cause of most of the other eye troubles is also the habit of staring.

Poor health and bad sexual habits are also supposed to be the cause of myopia but this is not so. These things can increase the strain if it already exists in the person or can produce a tendency to strain. Many persons having bad health or having bad sexual habits do not suffer from myopia or other eye diseases. There are many others who have very good health and lead sane lives and yet suffer from myopia or other eye diseases.

Treatment: — The remedy is not to avoid either near work or distant vision, but to get rid of the mental strain which underlies the imperfect functioning of the eye at both points; and it has been demonstrated in thousands of cases that this can always be done. The eyes are made to see with, and if when they are open they do not see, it is because they are under such a strain and have such a great error of refraction that they cannot see. The eye should be trained to focus correctly by central fixation, and to use themselves properly.

Eye Education by Central Fixation

Central Fixation: — The retina of the eye has a point of maximum sensitiveness called the "macula lutea" in medical terms. The eye with normal sight, therefore, sees that part of everything best on which it fixes itself, and the other parts not so well. This quality of the eye is called central fixation. Central fixation educates the eye to focus correctly. Central fixation is found defective in almost all abnormal conditions of the eye.

To improve central fixation it is necessary to take the help of a Snellen Test Card. Take the card in your hand. Keep your sight just below the letter 'C' on the white background. While keeping the sight below the letter, the whole of 'C' is visible but the bottom part of 'C' appears more distinct than the top part of 'C'. Now shift your sight to the white background just above 'C' and note that the top part of 'C' has become more distinct than the bottom part. In this way shift your sight three times from bottom to top and top to bottom of 'C'. Similarly practise on the smaller letters up to the sixth or seventh line of the Snellen Test Card. If the part of the letter regarded does not appear best, close the eyes for half a minute and remember the black or white colour, then open the eyes and practise on the letter. Then increase the distance of Snellen Test Card to 2, 3, 4, 5, 6, 7, 8, 9, 10 feet gradually and practise central fixation. While practising central fixation, palming may be done at times. If you find difficulty in regarding one part of a letter best, regard one letter of a line in such a manner that the one following it appears less distinct.

To improve central fixation on the reading matter of a book, keep the sight just below the line of letters and shift the sight from one end of the line to the other. Note that each word coming nearer the sight appears more distinct than the others. Blink gently.

Proper Use of the Eyes

Eyelids: — Eyelids play a great part in vision. The upper eyelids should remain downward, keeping the eye half-open. While looking upwards or in front the upper lids should not be raised, but only the chin.

It is very important for myopic patients to keep the lids in the right position.

Blinking: — The greatest things are always the simplest. The act of blinking is the first and simplest, and a most important action of the eyelids. In blinking the upper eyelid comes a little downwards to cover the pupil and is again raised. Wrong blinking is usually very irregular and jerky. Blinking is a quick method of resting the eyes and can be done unconsciously all the day long irrespective of what one may be doing. It is interesting to observe the blinking demonstration.

Look at any letter. Stop blinking, note that the blackness of the letter begins to fade. Now blink and note that the blackness reappears.

See how the eyelids work in a baby who has not yet lost its natural impulse and acquired the vicious habit of staring. You should blink at least 10 times a minute.

Reading: — Keep the book at a lower level than the chin so that the lids may not be raised. Then blink twice at least in reading one line. Do not read in the sun because the glare reflected from the paper causes strain to the eyes. Reading while lying can also be done without any discomfort, but you should keep the head raised and blink frequently. It is a great mistake to stop blinking while reading.

Fine Print: — Fine print reading is supposed to be one of the necessary evils of civilization, but the reading of fine print, when it can be done without discomfort, has invariably proved to be beneficial, and the dimmer the light in which it can be read, and the closer to the eyes it can be held, the greater the benefit. By this means severe pain in the eye has been relieved in a few minutes or even instantly. The reason is that fine print cannot be read in dim light and close to the eyes unless the eyes are relaxed, whereas large print can be read in good light and at ordinary reading distance although the eyes may be under a strain. When fine print can be read under adverse conditions, the reading of ordinary print under ordinary conditions is vastly improved. Reading fine print daily prevents and cures presbyopia (old-age sight) and many other diseases of the eye which usually occur in old age. Reading of fine print in candle light without or with glasses is very useful.

Seven Truths of Normal Sight

1. Normal Sight can always be demonstrated in the normal eye, but only under favorable conditions.
2. Central Fixation: The letter or part of the letter regarded is always seen best.
3. Shifting: The point regarded changes rapidly and continuously.
4. Swinging: When the shifting is slow, the letters appear to move from side to side, or in other directions with a pendulum-like motion.
5. Memory is perfect. The color and background of the letters or other objects seen, are remembered perfectly, instantaneously and continuously.
6. Imagination is good. One may even see the white part of letters whiter than it really is, while the black is not altered by distance, illumination, size, or form, of the letters.
7. Rest or relaxation of the eye and mind is perfect and can always be demonstrated.
When one of these seven fundamentals is perfect, all are perfect.

Specimen of Fine Print

Reading in Moving Vehicles: — Persons who wish to preserve their eyesight are frequently warned not to read in moving vehicles; but since under modern conditions of life many persons have to spend a large part of their time in moving vehicles, and as many of them have no other time to read, it is useless to expect that they will ever discontinue the practice. Fortunately the theory of its injuriousness is not borne out by the facts. When the object regarded is moved rapidly, strain and lowered vision is at first always produced; but this is temporary, and ultimately the vision is improved by the practice.

Writing: — While writing keep the sight on the point of the pen and move your sight with its movement, and blink frequently. A common mistake is to write forward and at the same time to look at the back letters.

Sewing: — Many women suffer from eye strain while sewing or doing needle work. They generally get a headache after working even for a short time. The mistake they commit is that they keep their eyes fixed on their work and blink at long intervals. They should blink frequently and move the eyes with the movement of the needle. If the needle comes up, the eyes also should move up and when the needle goes down to the cloth, the eyes should shift to the cloth. The shifting relieves the strain.

Cinema: — Cinematographic pictures are commonly supposed to be very injurious to the eyes, and it is a fact that they often cause much discomfort and the lowering of vision. They can, however, be made a means of improving the eyes. When they hurt the eyes, it is because the person strains to see them. If this tendency to strain can be overcome, the vision is always improved and if the practice of viewing pictures is continued long enough, many eye troubles are relieved.

How to see a Cinema Picture: — Sit erect comfortably, keep your upper lids down while raising the chin a little and blink frequently.

The common mistake, while seeing the cinema, is to keep the lids raised and stop blinking.

Sun Treatment and Palming

1. **Sun Treatment**: — The sun is a wonderful help in relieving all sorts of eye discomforts. Sometimes we get miraculous results. Everyone should do sun treatment.

Method of Sun Treatment: — Sit comfortably facing

the sun with closed eyes, and sway the body from side to side gently. One should continue for five to ten minutes. Morning or evening or when the rays of the sun are not keen, is the best time. One should stop sun treatment as soon as the sun causes discomfort. After enjoying the sun, one should come to the shade and wash the eyes with cold water to which 5 to 10 drops of OPHTHALMO may be added.

Eye wash is very effective in toning up the eyes. It gives relaxation. You may splash cold water on your eyes gently, or fill an eye-bath with cold water and put it against the eye in such a way that the lower margin of the eye-bath touches the lower eyelid, while the upper margin of the eye-bath remains free. Keep the eyes downwards and blink in the water of the eye-bath. Wash each eye for about a minute or two. Fixing the eye-bath against the eye and raising the head are not desirable.

2. **Palming**: — By palming I mean to close the eyes gently and cover them with the palms of the hands in such a way as to avoid any pressure on the eye-balls. When all the light is shut out by palming, one should experience a perfect dark before the eyes as if one were in a perfectly dark room. If it is not a perfect dark before the eyes during palming and some other colours appear, it indicates that the eyes and mind are under a strain. To relieve this strain imagine something perfectly black or some pleasant object like a flower, a boat floating on the river, clouds moving in the sky, etc. Some persons like to remember familiar things: thus a knife is remembered by a surgeon, dollies by girls, babies by mothers. When the imagination is perfect and corresponds to the reality, one sees a perfect dark before the eyes when they are closed and covered.

Palming may be done for two to five minutes or longer. You

may rest the elbows on the table or tuck a cushion below them.

After palming, open the eyes and practise central fixation on the Snellen Eye Testing Chart if your distant sight is defective; and on the reading test type if your near vision is defective. In most of the cases the benefit comes at the first sitting. Continue for some time to make the improvement permanent. For further directions, please read the book *Mind and Vision*.

White Line: — The white space in between the lines of print is called the white line. Look at the white lines of fine print of the reading test type, 'Fundamentals', of this book or look at the white lines of fine print. Shift your sight on the white line just below the line of letters, from one end to the other. Blink gently at each line. Make no effort to see the letters. It may be observed that the letters above the white line appear more distinct than before. If the letters are visible, the mind will automatically read them but an effort to look at the letters should not be there.

Practice of white line improves the reading sight and relieves the pain and discomfort of the eye.

Long and Short Swing: — Long swing is a great help to relieve discomforts and enables a person to adopt short swing. Long swing induces good sleep while short swing helps to improve the sight. When the swing is less than an inch, it is called short swing. It may be practised fifty to one hundred times.

Long Swing: — Stand with the feet about 12 inches apart, turn the body to the right — at the same time lifting the heel of the left foot. Do not move the head or eyes or pay any attention to the apparent movement of stationary objects. Now place the left heel on the floor, turn the body to the left, raising the heel of the right foot. Alternate.

Long Swing before bars of a Window: — Stand with the feet about one foot apart, move the body like a pendulum to the right while raising the heel of the left foot; then move the body to the left while raising the heel of the right foot. Alternate fifty to one hundred times.

Do not try to fix the gaze on the bars or on the background. Keep the sight shifting along with the movement of the head and blink at each side. Observe that the bars appear to move in the opposite direction.

Prevention of Myopia in Schools

Defective eyesight is found in most school children, and all attempts have failed to prevent myopia.

You cannot see anything perfectly unless you have seen it before. When the eye looks at an unfamiliar object it always strains more or less to see that object, and an error of refraction is always produced. When children look at unfamiliar writings or figures on the blackboard, distant maps, diagrams, or pictures they become myopic, though their vision may be under other circumstances absolutely normal. The same thing happens when adults look at unfamiliar distant objects. When the eye regards a familiar object, however, the effect is quite otherwise.

This fact furnishes us with a means of overcoming the mental strain to which children are subjected by the modern educational system. It is impossible to see anything perfectly when the mind is under a strain, and if children become able to relax by looking at familiar objects, they become able sometimes in an incredibly brief space of time, while to maintain their relaxation looking at unfamiliar objects.

Practice on the Snellen Test Card: — Place the Snellen Test Card upon the wall of each class-room. Everyday, children should read silently the smallest letters they can see from their seats, with both eyes together and then with each eye separately covering the other eye with the palm of the hand but avoiding any pressure upon the eye-ball. Fix a period of five minutes for it in the beginning of school work. The practice of five minutes daily is sufficient to improve the sight of all children in one week and to cure defective eyesight after some time.

Medical Examination of the Eye

When you are called for the eye examination, remember three points.

1. To cover one eye with the palm and not with the fingers. The fingers cause pressure on the eye-ball, and consequently the sight becomes defective. You are unable to read the smaller letters with that covered eye.

2. To keep the chin a little raised, and the lids down.

3. To blink gently on each letter.

Many students are disqualified from services and examinations due to defective eyesight. A good number of such men have passed the medical test after undergoing a course of treatment.

Superstition and Eye Education

Reading fine print is commonly supposed to be harmful to the eyes, and reading print of any kind in dim light and close to the eyes is regarded as a dangerous practice. Due to such a belief a student suffered a lot. He had pain in the eyes and pain in the head, he was in a state of agony and lost his peace of mind and his health. In the light of these superstitions, the facts contained in the following letter are particularly interesting:

"It happened frequently that I broke the glasses of my father when I was young. I was always scolded and punished. But one thing I used to ask my father, "Could you not do without glasses?" and my father always replied, "No." But how could my young mind be satisfied with my father's answer? My curiosity grew. I tried to get a satisfactory answer many times but in vain.

"I grew older and wiser and I was very strong in mathematics. I was fifteen, hale and harty, and continued to study hard. But a time came when I could not study, my eyes were strained and I never knew the cause. I realised that the eyes were getting weak. I went to the doctor and he treated me with eye-drops for a few days and I became all right. But the state of comfort could not continue long and the strain in the eyes grew worse. This time I went to Madras and a famous optician prescribed a pair of glasses and said, "Your eyes are in such a state that you must wear glasses if you want to progress well." I gave the least importance to his advice. His instruction revived my past memory and I repeatedly asked myself, "Could I not do without glasses?" I grumbled, "Oh, I am only sixteen and now I have to wear glasses! No, I shall not." And from that day I started hating them. But this did not solve my problem. I suffered a lot.

"Many months passed. I studied with pain in the eyes and pain in the head. I grew weaker in mathematics and lost my health, many worries cropped up in my mind. The condition of my mind and eyes became worse and worse. There was unbearable headache and I could not concentrate on my studies at home or school. I could not play either. I had lost my peace of mind. I observed that the pain increased while reading, specially when I was solving the problems of Geometry. It was at this time that I first learnt about Dr. Agarwal. I prayed to the Divine Mother for Her blessings and I got them. Next day at 8 o'clock I went to The School For Perfect Eyesight. Dr. Agarwal gave me a warm welcome. He asked some questions about my trouble and tested my eyesight on the Snellen Test Card and examined the eyes in the dark room. I observed more the Doctor's great interest in each patient than the process of testing the eyes. He gave me a few eye-exercises to do for three days only. To my great surprise the pain in my eyes was chased away and I was relieved from headache.

"Now I know why there was pain in my eyes. I used to read under high-power electric light, so after a short time the glare reflected from the paper used to cause pain in the eyes and head. I realised how soothing and helpful it was to read by candle light.

"The second thing which the Doctor advised me was not to stare at a thing. Formerly I used to stare at my Geometry figures constantly. I always thought that thus I was improving the power of concentration but it was not true. One should always blink gently every couple of seconds while studying or walking or doing anything else. In the beginning one has to do it consciously and wait until it becomes an unconscious habit. Thirdly, one should always be careful of the distance of the book from the eyes. One of my science-teachers told me to keep the book at about eighteen inches from the eyes but Dr. Agarwal instructed me to hold the book within twelve inches and he explained that the teacher must be over forty and so for him the greater distance suited.

"Lastly the Doctor opened my eyes to an important point. We all think that we should always read large print and that our eyes will never be spoiled by it. But it is a wrong notion. We must read small print. It is soothing and extremely beneficial for the eyes. We must blink twice while we read each line. It will relax not only the eyes but also the mind. These little truths were disclosed to me by Dr. Agarwal and now I have a great pleasure in exercising the eyes after five minutes' "palming". Palming refreshes the mind too.

"After the third day, I was in a state of serenity. And now I have convinced my father that one can do without glasses if one knows the right use of the eyes."

Relax and See

Vision is a process of mental interpretation of the retinal images. So in the act of seeing there is a close association between the mind and eyes. The eye without the mind will mechanically photograph the image but will not interpret it. The mind without the eye can imagine the images previously seen but will not tell you what is being photographed now. Correct seeing must be a perfectly co-ordinated action between mind and eye through Relax and See.

Relax and See is a quick effective process, of which most ophthalmologists are unaware. Hence their dogma of the incurability of errors of refraction such as myopia and hypermetropia continues. But now a number of doctors greatly appreciate the system of Relax and See and the time has come when its truth should be accepted by the medical profession for the welfare of humanity. How quickly the improvement in most of the cases of visual defects is achieved in the School for Perfect Eyesight is unimaginable. Here we give a short description to illustrate the subject.

The normal eye has three characteristics:

1. When the sight shifts from side to side of a letter, the letter appears to move in the opposite direction. This is Swinging.

2. The letter regarded appears clearest. This is Central Fixation.

3. The white centre of a letter appears whiter. This is Imagination.

These three characteristics are called normal illusions of the normal eye which are reduced or are absent in the defective eye. So to improve the vision it is necessary to develop the normal illusions.

The defective eye loses the frequency of shifting and becomes more or less immobile. Therefore mobility is essential. This mobility is to be developed by blinking education, long and short swing, game of ball, table-tennis, walking and observing the side objects moving in the opposite direction. By the creation of mobility discomforts of the eye fade away and one feels relaxed.

The defective eye loses the faculty of central fixation. It tries to see a large area at a time. So to develop central fixation adopt the following exercise; take the Snellen eye testing chart and shift the sight from top to bottom and bottom to top of a letter and observe two things:

a. When the sight shifts from top to bottom and bottom to top of the letter, the letter appears to move in the opposite direction.

b. The part of the letter regarded appears clearest.

The faculty of central fixation is also developed by reading fine print several times a day in good light and candle light. Myopic patients should avoid using glasses in reading and maintain relaxation by frequent palming and gentle blinking. By palming I mean: to close the eyes and cover them with the palms of the hands avoiding any pressure on the eyeballs; and to imagine something familiar and interesting.

To the defective eye the white centre of a letter does not appear whiter than the margin at varying distances. So there is loss of the imaginative faculty and the mind adds many other imperfections to the imperfect image received from the eye. So it is necessary to develop the faculty of interpretation of retinal images. This is achieved by imagination exercises:

a. Take the chart in hand and observe that the white centre of letter 'O' appears whiter at a distance where the sight is best. Gradually increase the distance. Or take two similar charts — one in hand and the other at five feet distance; look at the white centre on the near chart and then at the distant chart. Alternate.

b. Shift the sight on the white lines in between the lines of fine print. When the sight shifts from side to side, the lines of print appear to move in the opposite direction.

c. Take view-cards and develop the art of seeing as described in the book MIND AND VISION. The flatness of the picture will disappear and the three dimensional character of the picture will increase its beauty and improve the vision.

If there is pain or discomfort, strain or headache or double vision in reading, it is an indication that the person tries to concentrate the sight on the black part and makes an effort to see consciously or unconsciously. Any sort of complaint in reading indicates a wrong way of reading. All these troubles can fade away by the methods of Relax and See.

Here is a case of a European lady who was on the verge of giving up reading. At the age of forty-three she had difficulty in reading so much so that even with a 200 watt bulb she found it difficult to read. The letters got messed up and she could not read for more than half an hour at a time. To put it in her own words: "After five days of exercises at the School for Perfect Eyesight while looking at the white lines in between the photographic type reduction, I suddenly realised that the letters were very clear and that I was able to read the whole page of the smallest print which was impossible before. From then onward I never got the experience of messed letters again; not even after three hours of reading and more at one time. There is no strain and tension in my head any more and I am practically relieved of all complaints."

A case of glaucoma was suffering from constant eye strain, frequent headache, gradual loss of sight, seeing halos around light, with tension increased in both the eyes. Pilocarpine drops did not give proper relief, he was advised by Bombay doctors to go under operation.

In such cases operation worsens the trouble. The source of increasing loss of sight and constant eye strain were his glasses. He was using quite high power, bifocals, at the age of fifty. When he started his treatment, he was explained three main fundamentals of treatment. It took sometime to train the eyes to blink properly. Glasses were completely discarded from the very beginning of treatment. The result in two months treatment was surprising. He could see well at a distance and could read fine print without glasses. All his discomforts faded away. To preserve the improvement he devotes sometime in his eye education.

Questions and Answers

Q: What do you mean by Anatomy and Physiology of the eye?

A: Description of the form of the eye is called Anatomy, description of the functioning of the eye is called Physiology.

Q: You advised me to use glasses when necessary. I thought you were totally against them.

A: In your case I found that the best way to help you was to advise the use of glasses for distance but their disuse in reading as the near sight was quite normal.

Q: My daughter aged 8 years has developed defective vision for distance as well as for near things. She often gets a headache. What do you advise?

A: She can become all right. Apply Resolvent 200 to her eyes and let her face the morning sun with closed eyes for a few minutes. Then she should practise Palming and run around a chair, bouncing a ball to the ground, then read the Eye Chart at 5 to 10 ft. She should be taught how to blink frequently.

Q: I am seventeen, my eyesight began to deteriorate when I was seven. Every year the number of the glasses increased too much so that now I use 9 in the right eye, and 5 in the left. Can my eyes be benefited?

A: Yes, the improvement will be evident in a week's time if you can follow the proper course of treatment.

Q: My teacher says that I don't blink but wink. How to get the habit of blinking?

A: Practise with concentration the simple rhythms of blinking. The following natural exercises may be employed:

1. Walk slowly step by step and blink gently at each step.
2. Play with a ball, move it from hand to hand. To follow

the movement of the ball the eyes will begin to blink in a normal way.

3. Take a book of small type, shift the sight on the white lines in between the lines of print, blink once or twice on each white line.

4. Take a mirror. Look at the right eye and then at the left, blink on each side. It will keep you aware of wrong blinking.

Q: Your treatment has done much good to my eyes, now I want to extend the benefit to others. Is there any course to learn, or do you impart training?

A: You can attend the four year medical course in Ophthalmic Science. This will be a sort of synthesis of Allopathy, Ayurveda, Homeopathy and Bates Nature cure. Its study will enable the student to practise as an eye specialist.

Q: What is accommodation?

A: When the eye focuses at 6 metres or more, it is said to be at rest. When it focuses at a nearer point, it is called accommodation. When the eye is out of focus, the condition is called 'error of refraction' and there is short sight (myopia) or long sight (hypermetropia) without or with change of the eyeball's curvature (astigmatism).

Q: How to read? Is reading while lying in bed harmful to the eyes?

A: Hold the book at a distance from where the print is seen best. Usually it is about 10 inches. Then while reading move the head a little from side to side and blink gently once or twice in reading each line. Do not read in the sun or under bright artificial light because the glare reflected from the paper causes strain in the eyes. Reading while lying can also be done without any discomfort; for that, keep the head raised and blink.

Q: My eyesight is all right but I often get a strain and a headache after reading. What do you advise?

A: Just measure the distance from the book to your eyes. It may be more than 10 inches. If so, correct it. Take a specimen of diamond type or fine print and read it daily in good light as well as in candle-light. By reading fine print the capacity to read ordinary print is vastly improved. Reading fine print daily cures many a discomfort of the eye and quickly relieves headache.

Q: You recommend:
1. *Reading fine print*
2. *Reading in candle-light*
3. *Reading at a close distance*
All these instructions are diametrically opposite to all that we have been taught from childhood. How will you explain this fact?

A: The people who tell you to read big print in good light at an arm's length are mostly over forty. At this age the capacity to read fine print, to read in candle-light, to read at a close distance is usually lost. And if such persons attempt to read fine print, the eyes are strained. But if they had developed the habit of reading fine print from an earlier age, they could have maintained good eyesight in old age and prevented their eyes from deterioration. Then their advice would have been different. I on my part would advise even these people to take up fine print. They will not be able to read it at first, but they will be benefited by simply moving the sight in between the lines of fine print on the white lines. Fine print reading helps the eyes to relax while large print causes strain because the eye tries to see a large area at a time.

Q: A friend advises me to do some gymnastic eye exercises, that is, while keeping the head fixed move the eye-balls in various directions. Can I practise such exercises for the improvement of my eyesight?

A: Usually such exercises cause great strain. The fundamental principle is to move the head and eyes together in the same direction.

CHAPTER III

FUNDAMENTAL PRINCIPLE OF TREATMENT

Do you read imperfectly? Can you observe then that when you look at the first word, or the first letter, of a sentence you do not see best where you are looking; that you see other words, or other letters just as well as or better than the one you are looking at? Do you observe also that the harder you try to see, the worse you see?

Now close your eyes and rest them, remembering some colour, like black or white, that you can remember perfectly. Keep them closed until they feel rested, or until the feeling of strain has been completely relieved. Now open them and look at the first word or letter of a sentence for a fraction of a second. If you have been able to relax, partially or completely, you will have a flash of improved or clear vision, and the area seen best will be smaller.

After opening the eyes for this fraction of a second, close them again quickly, still remembering the colour, and keep them closed until they again feel rested. Then open them once more for a fraction of a second. Continue this alternate resting of the eyes and flashing of the letters for a time, and you may soon find that you can keep your eyes open longer than a fraction of a second without losing the improved vision.

If your trouble is with distant vision instead of near vision, use the same method with distant letters.

In this way you can demonstrate for yourself the fundamental principle of eye education and relaxation.

Favourable Conditions

The vision of the human eye is modified in many ways when

the conditions are unfavourable to good sight. Unfavourable conditions may prevail when the light is not agreeable to the patients. Some patients require a very bright light and others get along much better in a poor light. Many cases are hypersensitive to light and suffer from an intolerance for light which is called photophobia.

While intolerance of light may be manifest in most cases from some diseases of the eyes, there are many cases in which the eyes are apparently healthy and in which photophobia may be extreme. (The cure for this condition is to have the patient sit in the sun with his eyes closed allowing the sun to shine on his closed eyelids as he moves his head from side to side.)

There are patients with good sight whose vision is materially improved when used in a bright light, as well as those with good sight whose vision improves when the eyes are used in a dim light. The patient should practise with the Snellen Test Card in a bright as well as in a dim light to accustom his eyes to all conditions.

The ability to perceive halos, or an increased whiteness, around letters or inside letters is a favourable condition. By using a card having a hole in it, it is possible for many patients to see an increased whiteness around a letter or inside the letter, which improves their vision for the letter. When a card with a hole is not used, one may be able to imagine a white halo around the inner or outer edge of the black part of the letter "O". When the card covers the black part of the letter "O", for instance, the white centre becomes of the same whiteness as the rest of the white page, which proves that it is the contrast between the black and the white which enables one to imagine the white halos.

Demonstrate

1. That the sun treatment is of an immediate benefit to many diseases of the eye.

Before the treatment, take a record of your best vision on the Snellen Eye Chart and on the Reading test type. Then sit in the sun with your eyes closed, slowly moving your head a short distance from side to side, and allowing the sun to shine directly on your closed eyelids. Forget about your eyes; just think of something pleasant and let your mind drift from one pleasant thought to another. Before opening your eyes, palm for a few minutes. Then test your vision and note the improvement.

2. That long swing improves the sight, relieves pain, fatigue and many other disagreeable symptoms.

Take a record of your best vision with both eyes together and each eye separately without glasses. Stand with the feet about one foot apart facing a blank wall. Turn the body to the left, at the same time raising the heel of the right foot. Now place the heel of the right foot on the floor in its usual position; then turn the body to the right, lifting the heel of the left foot.

The head and eyes move with the body; do not make an effort to see more distinctly stationary objects which are apparently moving. Practice this fifty to one hundred times, easily without making any effort. Notice that, after practising, the vision for the test card improves.

Candle Practice

When reading of fine print in candle light is properly done, it proves extremely beneficial. It relieves the discomforts of the head and eyes and strain and improves the sight in cases of hypermetropia, astigmatism, presbyopia, myopia, early cataract, and glaucoma and in cases of retinal diseases. The flame stimulates the retinal cells and improves the blood circulation and gives a feeling of comfort, rest and relaxation.

When one reads in bright electric light or in the sun, the glare reflected from the paper causes strain and fatigue, sometimes loss of sight due to the development of serious complications. But in candle light there is no reflection from the paper and the light is just sufficient to read.

Reading in candle light may be done without or with glasses. If one candle light is not sufficient, one may use two candles. While reading, if one shifts the sight on the white lines in between the lines of print with gentle blinking, the print becomes very black and legible. Reading large print is detrimental to perfect sight because the eye tries to see a larger area at a time and this disturbs the sensitiveness of the retina. Reading of fine print in good light and candle light alternately is very helpful.

Concentration on the candle flame while counting 100 respirations is another way of helping the eyes and mind. It may be noted that the sight is on the flame but the mind is absorbed in respirations; then there is no strain. Staring at the flame is not good, it may cause strain and discomfort or headache. In such cases two candles may be used by keeping them 9 inches apart; then the sight is shifted from one candle to the other with the gentle rhythm of inhalation and exhalation. After concentration one may do palming or practise the long swing. Concentration on candle flame is very useful in hypermetropia and presbyopia. It helps in dissolving the formation of early cataract and relieves the tension in glaucoma cases.

Useful Hints in Reading

1. Hold the book at a distance from where it is seen best, move the head and sight with gentle blinking on each line. Usually the distance is 10 to 12 inches.
2. Move the book forward and backward.
3. Observe that each word appears darker.
4. Shift the sight just below the lines of letters and read.
5. Look at the white spaces instead of the black letters.
6. Move the body forward and backward.
7. For reading in lying posture, blinking is necessary.
8. Reading in dim light with strain helps myopic patients.
9. Reading in moving vehicles is not harmful.
10. Reading in candle light is extremely beneficial.
11. Read Fine Print and chart at 10 ft. alternately.
12. Read a portion and look away.
13. Read with a card hole.
14. Stitch and read alternately.
15. Reading of photographic type reduction is very useful.

Mistakes in Reading

1. No blinking or wrong blinking.
2. Trying to see many words at a time.
3. Distance more than what is needed.
4. Trying to see black instead of glancing at white.
5. Strong light on paper.

Shifting

When the normal eye has normal sight it is at rest and when it is at rest it is always moving or shifting. Shifting may be done consciously with improvement in the vision, or it may be done unconsciously with impaired vision.

Shifting may be done correctly or incorrectly. A wrong way to shift is to turn the head to the right while the eyes are turned to the left, or to turn the head to the left while the eyes are turned to the right.

To improve imperfect sight by shifting, it is well to move the head and eyes so far away that the first letter of the chart or object is too far away to be seen at all clearly. Shifting from small letters to large letters alternately may be a greater benefit than shifting from one small letter to another small letter. Quite frequently the vision is decidedly improved by shifting continuously from one side of a small letter to the other side, while the letter is imagined to be moving in the opposite direction. When the shifting is slow, short, and easy, the best results in the vision are obtained. Any attempt to stop the shifting always lowers the vision. The letter or another object which appears to move is usually shifting a short distance — one half or one quarter of an inch. It is not possible to imagine any particular letter or another object stationary for a longer period than one minute.

While the patient is seated, benefit can be obtained from shifting, but even more benefit can be obtained when the shifting is practised while the patient is standing and moving the head and shoulders, in fact the whole body, a very short distance from side to side. Shifting the whole body makes it easier to shift a short distance and may explain why this method is best.

Circular Swing

One of the best methods of obtaining complete relaxation

of the eyes and mind is the practice of thumb movement.

Place the hand against an immovable surface or on the thigh. Place the ball of the thumb lightly in contact with the forefinger. Now move the end of the thumb in a circle of about one-quarter of an inch diameter. When the thumb moves in one direction, the forefinger should appear to move in the opposite direction, although in reality it is stationary, only the thumb is moving. Some times just moving the thumb does not succeed to bring good relaxation unless one can count one, three, five or more odd numbers, when the motion is downwards, and an even number when the thumb moves upwards. It is not necessary for the patient to watch the movement of of the thumb in order to keep up the practice.

While watching the movement of the thumb, remember something imperfectly. At once, the thumb movement becomes irregular or may stop altogether. Demonstrate that any effort no matter how slight, to see, remember or imagine, interferes with the movement of the thumb. The thumb is so sensitive to an effort or strain that the slightest effort is at once recorded by the motion.

While watching the movement of the thumb, remember something perfectly. Notice that the movement of the thumb is slow, short, continuous and restful, the relaxation is felt in all parts of the body.

Many patients have been successfully treated for pain, headache and defective eyesight by the correct practice of circular swing.

Imagination Essential to Sight

Vision is a process of mental interpretation. The picture which the mind sees is not the impression on the retina, but a mental interpretation of it. To the mind objects seen appear to be in an upright position, but the picture on the retina is upside down. When the sight is normal the margins and openings of black letters on a white card appear whiter than the rest of the card, but this, of course, is not the fact, the whole background being of the same whiteness. For example, look at the white centre of the letter 'O' and compare the whiteness of the centre of 'O' with the whiteness of the rest of the card. The whiter you can imagine the centre of 'O' the better becomes the vision for the letter 'O'. The perfect imagination of the white centre of 'O' means perfect imagination of the black, because you cannot imagine the white perfectly without imagining the black perfectly.

When the vision is imperfect the imagination is also imperfect. The mind, in short, adds imperfections to the imperfect retinal images. A great part of the phenomena of imperfect sight are, therefore, imaginary and not in any way to be accounted for by the derangement of the visual apparatus. To a patient of imperfect sight the letter of the Snellen Test Card may appear gray or blue or with white spots over it; or, it may be, the size of the letter may be seen smaller or bigger, or a distorted shape may appear. Many persons with defective vision see floating specks before the eyes especially when they look towards some bright surface.

It is a great relief to patients to learn that these appearances are imaginary, and it helps them to bring the imagination under control. As it is impossible to imagine perfectly without perfect relaxation, any improvement in the interpretation of the retinal images means an improvement in the conditions which have led to a distortion of those images. Hence relaxation is the cure for most eye troubles. There is no more effective method of improving the sight, therefore, than by the aid of the imagination, and wonderful results have been obtained by this means.

When the mind is able to remember perfectly any phenomena of the senses, it is always perfectly relaxed. The sight is normal, if the eyes are open; and when they are closed and covered so as to exclude all the light. One sees a perfectly black field. If you can remember the ticking of a watch, or an odour or a taste perfectly, your mind is perfectly at rest, and you will see a perfect black when the eyes are closed and covered. If your memory of a letter or an object is according to the reality, you would see nothing but black when the light was excluded from your eyes. When this imagination is maintained while the eyes are open, the vision is quickly improved.

A school boy with a high degree of myopic astigmatism could see only two lines of the chart from 10 feet distance. By the aid of his imagination he could read the normal line within a fortnight. He could imagine a small letter of the chart with eyes closed as well as eyes open.

A college student used to see floating specks before the eyes most of the time during the day. When it was demonstrated that they were unreal, he was completely cured with the help of relaxation.

A student had myopia and was using glasses since the age of ten. Somehow the strain in the right eye increased so much that the colour, size and form of objects regarded altered. The straight things appeared curved and distorted. He was explained that most of the imperfections in his eyesight were due to eye strain, hence imaginary. He got great relief from these imaginary imperfections as soon as he learnt how to control the mind by eye education and mental relaxation.

In fact most of the blindness amongst civilized people is due to eye strain and mental strain and much of it is curable by the proper use of the eyes and mental relaxation.

Optical Illusions

Superficial vision is something like seeing the newspaper in the morning: the eye tries to see a large area, many words, at a time, and thus central fixation is disturbed.

As there is a superficial way of thinking and understanding there is a deeper way too, which gives deeper knowledge and sees the truth of everything.

Similarly there is a superficial way of seeing and deeper way of seeing. When one sees in a deeper way, it reveals the truth of the thing and the vision becomes free from imperfect illusion. Imperfect illusion is falsehood. But by training of the art of seeing the deeper perception of things can develop.

When deeper sense perception and deeper mind are active, the outer vision of things becomes more beautiful and attractive. In deeper vision of things there is no effort to see anything, it is perfectly effortless seeing.

By deeper way of seeing three dimensional character develops and along with that central fixation, imagination and swinging also develop.

Just use the eye like a camera without any effort, that will give you the idea of deeper way of seeing.

At the first glance there is always a strain to see, then if the eyes see without effort, deeper perception develops which sees a sort of reality.

If the reality of a thing is distorted and gives an impression of an illusion, it is called illusion of imperfect sight. But when the reality adopts more prominency and appears more beautiful, then it is an illusion of perfect sight. For example, 'O'; if it appears darker and its background whiter, then it is a normal illusion; but if 'O' appears gray and distorted and its white centre less white, then it is an imperfect illusion.

Our vision is illusion, that is, vision of the object depends on the mind's interpretation. All things when first seen give the impression of imperfect illusion, later when the eye adopts right way of seeing, the reality develops.

Deeper perception of things is also called piercing sight.

In the superficial way of seeing the eye tries to see the object, tries to get the impression of the objects, all at a time. When the object is regarded in a natural way without any effort to hold the object, the impression comes in detail and in a more perfect way.

When there is an optical illusion — a straight thing appears curved — it is an indication of superficial way of seeing; the person has lost central fixation at that moment. But if the same thing is seen with a deeper perception, the reality of the line will appear.

Perfect imagination of a black dot will give the sense of deeper perception, then the false illusion will fade away.

All optical illusions, imperfect or perfect, are an indication that what we see is mind's interpretation and this interpretation varies from person to person. If a portrait is made by seven artists, they all will differ in their expression due to the difference in their individuality.

For perfect seeing the organ must be perfect, the way of seeing must be perfect, the power of interpretation must be perfect.

Relief from Blindness

While many persons are benefited by the accepted methods of treating defects of vision by glasses and operations, there are some cases, known to every eye specialist, which get little or no help from them. These patients sometimes give up the search for relief in despair, and sometimes continue it with surprising pertinacity, never being able to abandon the belief that somewhere in the world there must be someone with sufficient skill who could cure them. The rapidity with which these patients respond to treatment by relaxation is often dramatic, and affords a startling illustration of the superiority of the relaxation methods to treatment by glasses and injections.

One case was a woman of thirty-five, a mother of five children, and her imperfect sight was accompanied by misery, insomnia and night blindness. Two years back there was robbery in her house and she was beaten. Since then this patient developed a great fear, lost sleep and the vision deteriorated; afterwards the condition became so serious that she was totally blind after 5.30 p.m. She went to various eye specialists of Orissa but found no relief. However, she did not waste time when she came to know about the SCHOOL FOR PERFECT EYESIGHT at Pondicherry. Her husband being a railway servant could easily travel and one morning I found the couple waiting to consult me. When examined, her vision proved fairly good in normal light, but in dim light she could not see anything. Various relaxation eye exercises were given and the eyes were bandaged for an hour twice a day. On the fifth day the husband reported that she could see all right in the evening. To test her ability to see in dim light I called them to my room after 6 p.m. she could see everything quite well in dim light as well as in electric light. It was now 7 p.m. Her husband suddenly pointing at something, asked her, "Do you see that?" She began to stare badly and lost her eyesight; she was then blind within five minutes. So the husband was warned not to test her in this way. After that she was left free. And now with two weeks' treatment she is quite all right at night, sleeps well, sees movies and remains cheerful.

Another was a case of blindness. The patient writes his experience:

"In 1954, one fine morning I suddenly noticed that I was seeing nothing practically with my right eye even with glasses. I consulted two leading eye specialists of Calcutta who after extensive treatment for about two months gave the verdict — 'Your right eye should be taken as lost.' After some time I had similar trouble with my left eye.

"I gave up all hope about my right eye as it had some retinal degeneration and I took it to be my fate that I should have to lead my life almost like a blind man. Then in December of that year Dr. Agarwal was on a short tour in Calcutta. I came in contact with him and underwent treatment by his unique method. After scrupulously following his directions for some weeks, I began to regain my lost vision. Within a very short period I went back to my normal life.

"Sixteen long years have passed and even today I can read and write without glasses and can move around the busy streets. My words are too inadequate to express my gratitude to Dr. Agarwal. But for him I would have been a blind man. Through him the Mother's Grace has been showered on my eyes."   A. S. Datta

This patient has still retinal degeneration in his right eye but that eye maintains almost normal vision and is far better than the other eye which has no degeneration and apparently quite normal. An eye specialist friend of his was surprised to observe this fact. The patient then put some questions to Dr. Agarwal.

Q: How is it that I maintain such a good vision although the centre of sight, the macular area, is still in a bad condition?

A: When there is some organic defect, there is always some functional defect, we have cured the functional defect, hence the sight has improved. Moreover, the macula is a small spot of the retina which is damaged, the rest of the retina is quite all right and Nature has helped the eye to function well through the rest of the retina.

Q: *It means patients suffering from semi-blindness due to retinitis, retinitis pigmentosa or some other retinal defect can also be benefited.*

A: Yes, most of them can be greatly benefited by eye education and mental relaxation. A case of retinitis pigmentosa showed remarkable improvement and was saved from blindness.

Questions and Answers

Q: *My eyes are sensitive to light, what should I do?*

A: Every morning for a few minutes face the sun with eyes closed while moving the head and body from side to side.

Q: *Why is it bad for the eyes to look at the sign-boards in the market-place or in other busy places?*

A: Usually one looks at the sign-boards while in fast movement and this gives strain to the eyes. Also, the letters of the sign-board are quite big, the eye tries to see the big letters all at a time and in such an attempt loses central fixation.

Q: *I want to know something about the construction and functioning of the eye. And here how does Dr. Bate's view differ from the orthodox?*

A: Have you seen a photographic camera? There is a diaphragm with an opening, a lens and a film. The eye is like a camera but it is an animate camera; it has the iris with an opening called 'pupil', the lens and retina. You adjust the focus in a camera by a change in the length of the body; the eye also adjusts its focus by a change in the length of the eyeball, and this change is made by the action of the outside muscles called 'oblique muscles'. (According to the orthodox view the eye changes its focus for vision at different distances by altering the curvature of the lens; this theory is not able to stand experimental proof and clinical observation.) The outside muscles function under the control of the mind.

But in one respect there is a great difference between the camera and the eye. The film of the camera is equally sensitive in every part; but the retina has a point of great sensitiveness, called central spot or 'macula lutea'. The eye with normal sight sees best where it fixes itself. That is why the object or part of the object regarded appears best. This quality of the eye is called central fixation.

The images received on the retina are carried through a nerve, called 'optic nerve', to the back part of the brain where the mind interprets these images and vision is the result.

This act of seeing is passive. Things are seen just as they are felt, heard or tasted without effort on the part of the person. The eye with normal sight never tries to see, and the moment it tries to see it ceases to be normal.

Q: What are the discoveries of Dr. Bates regarding the prevention of myopia in schools?

A: Analysing this problem Dr. Bates made the following discoveries:

1. That when a child tries to see bad handwriting or

unfamiliar charts on the blackboard a mental strain was produced.

2. This straining at a distance of 10 to 20 ft. caused a temporary condition of myopia, and if continued over a period of time the strain became an unconscious habit with resultant permanent myopia.

3. When testing children's eyesight with the Snellen Test Card, some with imperfect sight showed an improvement if allowed to read the chart a second or third time.

4. This temporary improvement of vision led him to discover that if children read the Snellen Chart daily, then the vision was usually permanently improved. This is because when reading familiar letters at a distance the mind is relaxed, and this unconscious relaxation is carried over when looking at unfamiliar writing on the blackboard.

5. A teacher who wears glasses has a bad psychological effect on the children, as they imitate the habits and nervousness. This results in a higher percentage of children developing defective vision in his class.

Chapter IV

MYOPIA AND HYPERMETROPIA

It is evident that all persons conscious of imperfect sight have a mental strain. Myopia is caused by a strain or an effort to see distant objects. It can always be produced in the normal eye temporarily by trying to see distant objects. Myopia is never continuous. At frequent intervals, lasting for a fraction of a second or longer, the patient is conscious of flashes of better vision. It is also a fact that when the mind is at rest and the eyes relaxed by the memory of a letter or some other objects, the myopia is lessened or disappears. Every myopic person has to maintain a mental strain with all its discomforts, in order to maintain a degree of myopia.

These facts suggest successful methods of treatment. Since mental strain or an effort to see distant objects is the cause of myopia, mental relaxation or rest is followed by benefit. By closing the eyes for five minutes or longer while letting the mind drift from one thought or memory to another, slowly, easily and continuously, rest of mind is obtained, and when the eyes are opened, the vision is usually improved for a short time, or for a flash.

Myopic patients can always demonstrate that closing the eyes and covering them with the palm of one hand or with those of both hands for half an hour always improves the distance vision temporarily. They are temporarily cured when their sight becomes normal at some distance; when they read fine print with perfect sight at four inches without glasses, they accommodate to just the same extent as a normal eye does when it reads perfectly at four inches.

Palming can only accomplish relaxation when the patient

does not try to see or imagine while palming. Some cases are able to palm more successfully than others. Some people can let their minds drift from one thing to another quite easily. A little girl was greatly benefited when the story of a black ant was told her. The black ant came out of the dark soil and climbed up the stem of a beautiful rose. It was slow work with the ant, but it kept on climbing, going on to the extremity of first one twig and then another, crawling to the extreme tip of every leaf until finally it located the flower. It crawled with great labour over the petals, until it found deep down in the centre of the rose a little white cup filled with honey. The patient could picture the ant carrying off some of the honey, crawling to the top of the flower, and then down back to the stem, finally meeting another ant on the ground. Then the second ant started off on the same journey.

The patient, while palming, listened very attentively to this talk which took about fifteen minutes. When she removed her hands from her closed eyelids, and opened the eyes, the vision was unusually good on the Snellen Eye Testing Card.

The story of the ant, with its successive mental pictures, suggests other stories of other things with other mental pictures, as a boat floating on a river with a varied scenery around. A mental trip to the seashore is also very restful when one imagines the waves flowing in and out.

When a hypermetropic patient fails to read perfectly at twelve inches or nearer, he usually feels the discomfort of mental strain. The hypermetropic eye can only read fine print perfectly when there is no mental effort. The vision of the hypermetropic eye is improved by the same methods which improve the vision of the myopic eye. Since the cause of hypermetropic is mental effort, its cure is obtained when the mental effort disappears.

In presbyopia the vision for the distance is usually good, while the ability to read at the near point fails. It is said that presbyopia begins soon after the age of forty and then gradually increases. It has been observed by many doctors that presbyopia may begin before the age of forty, or it may not appear until a much later date. I have seen patients over sixty years of age who had normal sight in each eye for the distance, and they could read small print at twelve inches. A popular belief is that presbyopia is due to the hardening of the lens. Dr. Bates has proved with facts that the lens is not a factor in accommodation, and that the cause of presbyopia is a mental strain when trying to see or read at a near point. Presbyopia is cured by practising relaxation methods. Presbyopic patients are greatly benefited when they imagine the white spaces in between the lines of print whiter than the margin of the page. The eyes, when reading perfectly, do not look directly at the letters, but at the white spaces or the halos.

Headache

Often headache is due to the wrong use of the eyes while reading, writing, sewing or seeing cinema. But such a headache is quite temporary and is usually not quite severe. Right education of the eyes will cure this kind of headache.

Severe headache is usually due to lack of mental relaxation. Many myopic patients get severe headache when they use the distant glasses for reading also. They are quickly cured by avoiding glasses in reading and by relaxation exercises and by reading fine print in dim light. A myopic patient was suffering from severe headache for ten years. Within a week he was perfectly all right by exercising mental relaxation and by avoiding glasses for reading. A boy suffering from severe headache for three months was cured by reading fine print in candle light and by reducing the distance of holding his book. A girl was suffering from constant headache for six years and had a pair of glasses and had no relief by any treatment. She was cured within a few days by correct palming.

Some patients complain of headache when they put on glasses. Usually the number is high in such cases. A lady was using plus glasses all the time. She often suffered from severe attacks of headache and dizziness. She was cured of headache by not using the glasses and by frequent palming.

Headache appearing after sleep is usually due to strain during sleep. Such cases are usually cured by light diet at night and by long swing and palming.

In some cases headache appears from sunrise to sunset and the headache is quite severe. Such cases are cured usually in a day by nasal drops which bring out sufficient nasal discharge.

Headache due to constipation, cold and fever needs medical treatment which should not be of suppressive type.

See Things Moving

When the sight is perfect the subject is able to observe that all objects regarded appear to be moving. A letter seen at the near point or at the distance appears to move slightly in various directions. The pavement comes toward one in walking, and the houses appear to move in a direction opposite to one's own. In reading, the page appears to move in a direction opposite to that of the eye. If one tries to imagine things stationary, the vision is at once lowered and discomfort and pain may be produced, not only in the eyes and head, but in other parts of the body too.

This movement is usually so slight that it is seldom noticed till the attention is called to it, but it may be so conspicuous as to be plainly observable even to persons with markedly imperfect sight. If such persons, for instance, hold the hand within six inches of the face and turn the head and eyes rapidly from side to side the hand will be seen to move in a direction opposite to that of the eyes. If it does not move, it will be found that the patient is straining to see it in the eccentric field. By observing this movement it becomes possible to see or imagine a less conspicuous movement, and thus the patient may gradually become able to observe a slight movement in every object regarded. Some persons with imperfect sight have been cured simply by imagining that they always see things moving.

The world moves. Let it move. All objects move if you let them. Do not interfere with their movement, or try to stop it. This interfering cannot be done without an effort which impairs the efficiency of the eye and mind.

Memory Swing

Memory swing is done with the eyes closed while one imagines himself to be looking first over the right shoulder and then over the left shoulder, while the head is moved from side to side. The eye-balls may be seen through the closed eyelids to move from side to side in the same direction as the head is moved.

The memory swing can be shortened by remembering the swing of a small letter, a quarter of an inch or less, when the eyes are closed.

The memory swing has given relief in many cases of imperfect sight from myopia, astigmatism, and inflammations of the eye-ball. It may be practised incorrectly, just as any other swing may be done wrong, and then no benefit will be obtained.

Recall to memory the letter O of small type and shift your attention from side to side of O and observe that the letter O appears to move in the opposite direction. This motion, when the shifting is done properly, is very short, less than the width of the letter.

Now do the same with a letter on the test card. If the shifting is normal, it will be noted that the letter appears to have a slight motion. Do not attempt to concentrate, otherwise the swing will stop and the blackness of the letters of the chart will become dim.

Mental Pictures

With imperfect sight, a mental picture of one known letter of the Snellen test card is seldom remembered, imagined or seen perfectly when regarded with the eyes open. By closing the eyes, the same mental picture may be imagined more perfectly. By alternately imagining the known letter as well as possible with the eyes open and then remembering it better with the eyes closed, the imagination improves the vision and unknown letters are seen with the eyes open. It is a fact that a good or perfect imagination of mental pictures brings about a measure of improvement in eyesight which is convincing.

While the colon is a valuable punctuation mark, its mental picture is very valuable to help the memory, imagination and sight. With the eyes closed or open, the top period should be imagined best while the lower period is more or less blurred and not seen so well. In a few moments it is well to shift the sight and imagine the lower period best while the upper period is imagined not so well. Common sense makes it evident that one period cannot be imagined best unless there is some other period or other object which is seen worse. The smallest colon that can be imagined is usually the one that is imagined more readily than a larger colon. To remember or imagine a colon perfectly requires constant shifting. When the colon is remembered or imagined perfectly, and this cannot be done by any effort or strain, the sight is always improved. One may feel that the memory of a very small colon should be more difficult than the memory of a large one, but strange to say it can be demonstrated in most cases that the very small colon is remembered best.

Glaucoma and Stare

When a patient stares, an effort is always made to hold the eyes still without moving them. It is impossible to hold the eyes perfectly still. Trying to do the impossible always requires strain. This strain can be demonstrated to be a mental strain. With a mental strain, the memory and imagination becomes imperfect and imperfect sight results. Pain, fatigue, dizziness, are acquired or made worse.

Glaucoma, acute or chronic, has been produced by the stare. Most common symptoms of glaucoma are hardness of the eye-ball, contraction of the nasal field, appearance of a halo around lights. The look of the glaucoma patient is a clear indication of the stare. Such patients use the stare to improve their vision and are unconscious that an effort to see is being made. So it is good to teach these patients how to stare and how to relax. By staring the patient then becomes conscious that it affects the sight and increases the tension, while by relaxation the severity of the glaucoma symptoms is lessened.

Many adults past middle life unconsciously stare and produce glaucoma. By practice they become conscious of the stare. When the stare is strong enough and sufficiently prolonged, it increases the hardness of the eye-ball. In the matter of treatment the great problem is to suggest measures which will enable the patient to demonstrate that the stare is the cause of increased tension of the eye-ball in glaucoma.

When the forefinger of one hand is held about six inches to one side of the face and about six inches straight ahead, the patient, by moving the head and eyes from side to side slowly or rapidly, can imagine the movement of the finger from side to side. This movement of the finger is called variable swing. When the finger appears to move, the injurious stare is prevented.

Prolonged palming and long swing alternately also prove very helpful to break the habit of staring. One should learn to blink at each step while walking and imagine the side objects moving backwards. Two candles may be put one foot apart, and the patient shifts the sight from one candle flame to the other, then the candle flames appear to move in the opposite direction.

Sun treatment proves effective in glaucoma. The patient faces the sun with the eyes closed and moves a ball from one hand to the other. While moving the ball in this way he shifts his eyes and head from side to side.

Condensing the rays of the sun on the white part of the eye-ball is very effective in chronic cases of glaucoma. While facing the sun the patient is directed to look as far down as possible, and in this way the pupil is protected by the lower lid. Then by gently lifting the upper lid, only the white part of the eye is exposed, while the sun's rays strike directly upon this part of the eye-ball. The sun glass may then be used on the white part of the eye. Care should be taken to move the glass from side to side quickly. The length of time devoted to focussing the light on the white part of the eye is never longer than a few seconds.

If the patient is not totally blind due to glaucoma, then in almost all cases the vision improves by relaxation treatment. Cases of early symptoms of glaucoma are cured quickly, sometimes within a few days. In such cases shifting the sight on the white lines of fine print proves very effective. When patients can read fine print comfortably without or with glasses in good light and in candle light, they are quickly relieved of glaucoma symptoms. The pain and discomfort is chased away. It is because fine print cannot be read by strain; one can read it well only by relaxation.

A lady patient had developed the habit of strain and often suffered from the pain and discomfort of glaucoma. Her one eye was operated upon for glaucoma but there was no relief, the condition grew worse and worse. Her pain was completely cured and the vision considerably improved by sun treatment and relaxation. The orbital swing helped a great deal in her treatment.

Orbital swing: Move the index finger in the air in a circular way, follow the movement of the finger while moving the head and eyes with eyes closed. It seems as if the eye-ball is rolling in the orbit. When done properly, it brings quick relief from pain in the eye-balls.

Hypermetropia

Persons who need plus glasses suffer from hypermetropia. Hypermetropia is found developing at any age but it becomes a great puzzle to the doctor when hypermetropia is found developing in old age when the lens becomes hard. Recently within a week five persons who developed hypermetropia in their old age were recorded in our Eye Clinic. At first these persons needed glasses only for reading at the age of forty but later on they were prescribed bifocals. Then, due to strain in reading, number of glasses went on increasing quite fast. In the case of a lady patient the last prescription of glasses was of +4.0 for distance and +7.0 for reading, and even with such a high power of glasses the vision was quite poor and she was suffering from headache and eye strain. These cases drew our attention to study hypermetropia more carefully.

When the sight is good for distant vision that does not mean that the sight is also good for reading at ten or twelve inches. Poor sight for reading is usually corrected by the use of reading glasses. In old age serious eye troubles are caused by the strain of hypermetropia. In the early stage these diseases are more readily curable than after they have become chronic and more serious. The treatment which cures hypermetropia is the treatment which prevents and cures serious eye diseases. The strain of hypermetropia causes glaucoma; when this strain is relieved, glaucoma usually improves.

In studying the production of hypermetropia it is interesting to note the conclusion of a well known eye specialist. He was asked this question: "Is hypermetropia curable?" He replied that it was not curable. He was then asked, "Why do you claim that no one can cure hypermetropia?" He answered, "I know that it cannot be cured because I was unable to succeed and if I cannot succeed no one else can."

A patient reported that he was using plus bifocals for a long time but after his retirement he gave up reading and did not use glasses also. This improved his eyesight greatly. When tested on the eye chart he could read the last but one line from 10 ft. and could read fine print in good light at 12 inches. When he reported this fact to his optician, the latter did not believe his statement. When patients of hypermetropia improve their eyesight spontaneously or by relaxation treatment, the result becomes a very great puzzle to the doctors and opticians. It is because their whole conception about the formation of visual defects is based on fallacies; they cannot answer this question: why is hypermetropia developed or cured in old age? And when such cases come before them, the tendency is just to ignore and give suitable glasses.

Children suffering from hypermetropia are very easily cured by palming and reading of the Snellen Eye Chart and fine print daily. All their discomforts fade away within a few days and their memory and imagination improve. A child wearing glasses of +6 was cured in a week's time.

A patient of hypermetropia was developing a cataract; by the treatment of hypermetropia the cataract was cured and all the discomforts of reading faded away. In another case hypermetropia changed into myopia when he was fifty-seven. He had practised some Yogic exercise of concentration on a bright object.

Questions and Answers on Hypermetropia

Q: What is hypermetropia?

A: The other name for hypermetropia is farsight although the vision is not clear either for distance or for near. Why? Because in hypermetropia the eye-ball is too short from the front backward, and the rays of light coming from distant objects and near objects are focussed behind the retina and not on the retina.

Q: Is hypermetropia a permanent condition?

A: Hypermetropia is not a permanent condition and this

fact is evident from the various prescriptions of glasses which the patient gets from the doctors. Though the orthodox view is that hypermetropia is a permanent condition from birth, the fact is that hypermetropia is acquired at any age.

Q: What are the symptoms of hypermetropia?

A: Usually the eyes are tired soon in reading, or one finds difficulty in reading some small print. Strain and feeling of pain and headache also are quite frequent. At times the letters of a book appear double or read wrongly. It is hypermetropia which causes many complications in the eyes in old age, as cataract, glaucoma, diseases of the optic nerve and retina. Therefore it is necessary to treat hypermetropia at least to relieve the discomforts and to prevent serious complications. Fortunately the treatment of hypermetropia is easier than of myopia and usually hypermetropic patients are greatly benefited in a short time.

Q: It is often seen that hypermetropia is cured or lessened spontaneously. How does it happen?

A: According to the orthodox view it is not permissible to suppose that there has been a change in the shape of the eye-ball. Therefore, when hypermetropia disappears or is lessened we are asked to believe that the eye, in the act of vision, both at the near point and at the distance, increases the curvature of the lens sufficiently to compensate, in whole or in part, for the flatness of the eye-ball. But according to the discoveries of Dr. W.H. Bates hypermetropia is relieved by the relief of the strain on the eye and the eye-ball is elongated by relaxation treatment.

Q: I had good eyesight at one time but due to proof reading in dim light my eyesight suffered and now I use plus bifocals, and the number goes on increasing almost every year. How?

A: According to the orthodox view there is no explanation for this increase in the number of glasses because the lens becomes hard in old age. But according to Dr. Bates hypermetropia is caused by a strain in near work. Due to such a strain the rectus muscles contract and shorten the eye-ball.

Q: Can hypermetropia be produced in the normal eye if strain is the cause?

A: When the normal eye reads in dim light with strain, hypermetropia is produced. But if the myopic eye reads in dim light with strain, myopia is decreased and the vision for distance is improved.

Q: How is the strain caused in near work?

A: By reading under high power of electric light or in dim light; by staring at near point and no blinking; haste in reading; by reading bigger and unfamiliar writings, etc.

Q: What is the best preventive for hypermetropia?

A: Reading of fine print with gentle blinking without or with glasses, and concentration on a candle flame while counting 100 respirations.

Q: What is the treatment for hypermetropia?

A: Palming, swinging, shifting the sight on white lines in between the lines of fine print and reading of the Snellen Eye Chart placed in dim light at a twenty ft. distance. The editor of *Mother India*, Mr. Sethna, has discarded his plus bifocals after using them for about 20 years and can read fine print.

Q: If some patients are not cured by the relaxation treatment, then what will you do?

A: When some persons are not able to rest their eyes sufficiently then I prescribe glasses also and tell them to do palming and read fine print with glasses.

Q: What precautions do you advise for a case of glaucoma in its early stage?

A: 1. Correct the habit of blinking.

2. Play with a ball, moving the ball from hand to hand. Shift the sight with the movement of the ball.

3. Concentration on two candle flames.

4. Read small print in good light and candle light alternately.

5. Often the prescription of glasses used by the patient is found high; better avoid glasses as far as possible and use correct glasses.

Q: What is the treatment for detachment of retina?

A: The habit of right blinking, frequent palming and reading of fine print is the sure preventive for detachment of retina.

Eye education and mental relaxation exercises will cure detachment of retina. Even if the operation is advisable, patient ought to be educated how to relax the eyes to prevent any further relapse.

CHAPTER V

TREATMENT OF MYOPIA

The cause of myopia is not reading small print but an effort to see distant objects. When the normal eye stares at a distant object or tries to read two parts of the Snellen Test Card letter perfectly at the same time, an effort to see is made and myopia is produced. There is a strain; and the greater the strain, the more imperfect the vision. This suggests the cure of myopia.

The production of improved or perfect sight is easy as it does not need any effort, it comes only by rest or relaxation. Most people with myopia are not conscious of the stare or strain or the effort to see. Persons with normal vision are often able to demonstrate that myopia is caused by strain.

In the treatment of myopia the first thing is that the patient should know that the cause of myopia is the stare or the effort to see at a distance. When the patient looks at the white centres of letters of the Snellen Test Card with gentle blinking and without any effort to see, the vision is always found to be improved, and when such a practice is continued several times a day, the patient is habituated to look at things without effort and the vision is considerably improved.

The Snellen Test Card can be used in various ways to improve the vision. Usually patients of myopia improve more when the chart is held at five feet or less, then the distance of the chart is gradually increased. When the patient sways his body from side to side, the chart appears to be moving in the opposite direction, and this imagination is beneficial. Then gradually the sway is shortened. If the test card does not appear to sway, it is usually an indication of strain or an effort to see.

If the letters on the test card appear double, it is because the patient is trying to see the letters. This double vision cannot happen if the patient imagines the card moving slightly from side to side and does not try to see the letters. Palming when done successfully relieves such symptoms quickly.

Reading newspaper type or fine print in dim light is very useful to myopic patients. It helps to lessen myopia and develop normal vision. Looking at a blank wall of one colour and imagining something interesting and pleasant is also very useful to all cases of defective vision.

If one can imagine a small letter "O" with its white centre perfectly, first with eyes closed, then with eyes open while glancing at the chart letters, the vision is decidedly improved and sometimes surprising results are obtained.

Reading fine print or photo type reduction in good light, in dim light and in candle light alternately helps the patients to relax their eyes; all pain and strain and headache are quickly relieved.

Control of relaxation is the key to cure myopia and many other diseases of the eye.

Before and after sleep practise palming. While walking or dressing or going to the school blink gently.

If you can teach others how to blink, this will greatly help you to adopt the right habit.

Before children go to the school, they should read the chart at ten or twenty feet distance and read fine print. By this practice many of their defects of vision have improved and their eyesight restored to normal.

The superiority of the relaxation treatment is very well indicated in a letter received from Mr. S. S. Parekh of Ahmedabad Advance Mills: "My two daughters, Hemangini and Surekha, who took eye treatment from you at Pondicherry were showering all praise on you for the wonderful effect it had on their eyes. The number of Surekha has completely disappeared and that of Hemangini has gone down more than 50%."

Variations in Eyesight

1. Usually myopic patients of -3 or more can hardly read more than 10/200, and can hardly read the small print of Fundamentals at more than 6 inches.

2. But some cases of high myopia can read 10/50 line or more without glasses and do not show much improvement with glasses. They can read small print at about 10 inches.

3. In some cases the vision is quite poor for distance though corrected with glasses but in reading they can read the small print at about 12 inches.

4. In a small number of cases once the glasses are prescribed, the number is almost constant. This is harmless myopia.

5. Mostly the number of glasses goes on increasing slowly, say once in two years a little increase.

6. In certain cases the deterioration in eyesight is quite fast. Such cases when timely treated respond well.

7. Usually the variation is quite marked when the patient looks at objects with lids raised and when lids down and blinking.

8. Some myopic patients feel great strain and headache as soon as they put on glasses while some are greatly relieved by the use of glasses.

9. Use of glasses in reading is usually detrimental because the vision for reading is quite good or better than with glasses.

10. All cases of visual defects improve their eyesight by eye education and mental relaxation. Flashes of great improvement are quite often.

11. In some cases the error or refraction as demonstrated

by retinoscope does not change though the vision is considerably improved and comes to normal with the lower power of glasses.

12. In a case of +8 hypermetropia the vision was almost the same with or without glasses. By eye education his vision greatly improved and he felt no necessity of glasses. But retinoscope continued to show the same error of refraction.

13. It is difficult to say who will respond much to the treatment though some idea is formed due to experience and inspiration. However, persons having -12 or more while going under treatment feel no difficulty without glasses in their movements; they walk about without strain, without headache.

14. A case of -7 using contact lenses greatly surprised us when she improved her eyesight to almost normal in 3 days. We had no idea that such a high myopic case could improve so much. This broke our old conception.

15. Two similar cases with equal vision without glasses require different power of glasses for full correction. First case needs -8 dioptres to see 6/6 — whereas the second one, with nearly the same history needs only -1.5 dioptres. According to the laws of optics such a queer phenomenon is not possible. Moreover, in the first case, after the treatment of his myopia, glasses of -6 dioptres made little difference. Without glasses he begins to see as much as what he used to see, prior to the treatment, with the glasses of -5.5 dioptres. Whereas in the second case addition of mere -0.5 makes a great difference though according to the laws of optics a lense of a certain dioptre will, in all conditions, have the same divergence faculty. And above all the retinoscope does not show much improvement though the subject experiences for sure.

Vision and Education

Poor sight is admitted to be the cause of retardation at school and it is commonly assumed that all disadvantages might be prevented by suitable glasses.

There is much more involved in defective vision, however, than mere inability to see the blackboard or to use the eyes without pain or discomfort. Defective vision is the result of an abnormal condition of the mind, the mind is under strain, and when the mind is under strain and is in an abnormal condition the process of education cannot be conducted with advantage. By putting glasses upon a child we may, in some cases, neutralize the effect of this condition and improve his mental faculties to some extent; but we do not alter fundamentally the condition of the mind, and by confirming it in a bad habit we may make it worse.

Among the faculties of the mind which are impaired when the vision is impaired is the memory; and unless the strain of the mind is relieved, very little will be gained by putting glasses on a child to see better. The extraordinary memory and keenness of vision of primitive people was due to the mind at rest. Perfect memory and perfect sight go together.

Under the present educational system there is a constant compulsion on the children to remember. This compulsion always fails. It spoils both the memory and the sight. We remember without effort, just as we see without effort, and the harder we try to remember or see, the less we are able to do so.

The sort of things we remember are the things that interest us, and the reason children have difficulty in learning their lessons is because they are bored by them. Boredom is a condition of mental strain which affects the memory as well as eyesight. The fundamental reason, both for poor memory and poor eyesight in school children, in short, is our irrational and unnatural educational system. Montessori has taught us that it is only when children are interested that they can learn.

When one is not interested, one's mind is not under control, and without mental control one can neither learn nor see. Not only the memory but all other mental faculties are improved when the eyesight becomes normal. It is a common experience with patients cured of defective sight to find that their ability to do their work has improved.

A teacher reported that one of her pupils used to sit doing nothing all day long and apparently was not interested in anything. After the eye testing card was introduced into the classroom and his sight improved, he became anxious to learn, and speedily developed into one of the best students in the class. In other words, his eyes and his mind became normal together. In another case symptoms of irritable temperament were quickly relieved when the vision became normal. It is always observed that when the sight is improved by relaxation methods, the faculties of the mind are also improved. Myopic patients, who use glasses all the time, often complain of loss of memory; when they learn how to rest the mind and avoid the use of glasses in reading, their memory is improved quickly.

From all these facts it is clear that the problem of education cannot be solved simply by putting glasses before the eyes of children. The children should be taught the right use of the eyes without effort or strain. They should be encouraged to read the Snellen Test Card daily with gentle blinking and do palming.

Besides the methods of mental relaxation, it is worth the trouble to teach children who have so-called incurable diseases how to enjoy themselves for long periods of time both winter and summer. Their eyes as well as their bodies are kept in motion while playing games or engaging in sports which relieve the stare and strain that cause imperfect sight. It is so much more efficient and better than drugs.

Unfamiliar objects always cause strain on the minds of children. Hence children learning to read, write, draw, or sew, always suffer from defective vision, because of the unfamiliarity of the lines or objects with which they are working. They can be helped by chart reading daily and by games which keep them in motion.

Eye Education

Eye education has been proved to be effective in preventing and improving defective vision in school children.

A Snellen Test Card was used for more than a year by a teacher as a means of preventing and improving defective eyesight. This card was placed on the wall of the classroom. Every day, while sitting quietly in their seats, the children were encouraged to read the Snellen Test Card, with each eye separately, covering one eye in such a way as to avoid pressure on the eye-ball. This required only a few minutes and did not interfere with the regular school work. The results obtained from this simple practice were very gratifying. Almost all the children were cured of their headaches and other discomforts and improved their sight to normal.

PALMING. Many children suffer from headaches, eye-strain and fatigue. When the eyes are closed and covered with the palms of both hands, it is possible to obtain rest and relaxation of the nerves of the eyes and of the body generally, provided the palming is done properly. Most children are fond of pleasant memories and when they palm, they usually think of pleasant things such as games, flowers etc. which help them to palm successfully. When school children learn by experience that palming is a benefit to their sight, headaches, nervousness, or other disagreeable symptoms, they will practise palming very frequently without being encouraged to do so.

SWAYING. Children should stand with their feet about one foot apart and sway the whole body from side to side. When this is practised, the stare, strain or effort to see is prevented and the vision is always improved.

FINE PRINT. When school children are able to read fine print at the distance from their eyes at which they see it best, the eye strain is relieved as fine print cannot be read with an effort. The distance where fine print is seen best varies with people. All children should not be encouraged to see fine print at the same distance from their eyes. Reading fine print in candle light proves extremely beneficial.

BLINKING. The normal eye, with normal sight blinks frequently, easily and rapidly, without effort or strain. If children do not blink frequently, but stare and try to see things with the eyes open continuously, the vision is always impaired. At first the child should be reminded to blink consciously but it soon becomes an unconscious habit and the vision is improved.

SWINGING. When the eyes move slowly or rapidly from side to side stationary objects, which are not regarded, appear to move in the opposite direction. The teacher can direct the children to stand beside their desks while swaying from side to side. The pupils can notice that the desks in front of them, the blackboard, and the Snellen Test Card are all moving in the direction opposite to the movement of their bodies. While walking children can notice that the floor appears to move towards them. If the children are conscious of the movement of the floor and other objects, the stare or strain is prevented, and the vision is always improved; but if they do not notice the movement of objects when they themselves move, they are apt to strain and the vision is lowered.

When children imagine the Snellen Test Card to be moving from side to side, the imagination of black letters or of the white spaces is improved. If the head and eyes are moved an inch or less from side to side, the Snellen Test Card and the letters on it will also appear to move an inch or less. With the aid of such a short swing, the vision is greatly improved. But if the letters do not appear to move, an effort is soon manifest. The children then find that trying to see a letter stationary requires a strain and is difficult. It seems strange, although it is true, that to fail to have perfect sight required an effort and hard work. In other words, perfect sight can only come easily and without effort; while imperfect sight is obtained with much discomfort and effort.

School Children

It is estimated that in big cities one tenth of the school children wear glasses and their defects go on increasing in spite of all care. It is believed by many that the cause of defective eyesight in school children is the use of small print in the text books. When some schools experimented to use only large print for the children, eye-strain and headache and other troubles became more numerous than when small print was employed; repeated trials of books in which large print was used always failed to prevent discomfort. Just as many children wore glasses after the use of text books with large print as when the books were printed in small print. Evidently, the cause of imperfect sight in school children was not connected in any way with the size of print used in text books.

It has been generally believed also that the imperfect light of school rooms is the cause of imperfect sight in school children. In fact, the amount of light has nothing to do with the cause of imperfect sight. Children with myopia or hypermetropia have been benefited or cured within a few weeks or earlier by eye education when a poor light or a bright light was used. They have been cured of their discomforts by reading very small print in good light as well as in candle light or poor light.

Dr. Cohn has done an enormous amount of work to determine the cause, prevention, or cure of imperfect sight in school children. He recommended what was considered to be the best form of lighting in schools and also devoted a great deal of his time to desks and seats. He believed that he had made a valuable discovery towards prevention of imperfect sight when he recommended an apparatus which prevented school children from leaning far forward when they were studying or writing. After his method had been in use for some time, the vision of children was tested. Much to the surprise of the parents of the children, the vision was not benefited. A friend asked Dr. Cohn for his statistics on children who were benefited; he said no children were benefited and that the method was a failure.

Dr. Bates has proved repeatedly through various experiments and clinical observations that any effort or strain to improve the vision always lowers the vision. Straining the eyes to see at long distances always produces nearsightedness or myopia. When efforts are made to see at the near point continuously, the eyes become far-sighted or hypermetropic. It can be demonstrated that the normal eye with normal sight becomes imperfect by a strain to see. When the eyes are relaxed the vision always becomes normal.

Dr. Bates recommends a system of eye education for the prevention and cure of imperfect sight in school children. A Snellen Test Card is used as a means to prevent and improve imperfect sight. Children suffering from defective vision may read it frequently and do palming.

A Case of Myopia and Nystagmus

A Report by a Patient's Father

Science has greatly progressed, man can land on the moon and news can spread all over the world in a minute. But what a pity that Ophthalmic Science seems to be two hundred years backwards. Almost every eye specialist believes that there is neither any preventive nor cure for defective vision. For such defects as myopia, hypermetropia and presbyopia they prescribe glasses and help the patients to see well but there are many cases where glasses fail to work as a palliative even. Any rational mind will think that science is yet in a backward stage. But there is one doctor in India who cures his patients of defective vision by means of education and mental relaxation.

My daughter Vijay Laxmi, aged ten years was semi-blind, she was suffering from nystagmus, that is, her eyes were making short movements from side to side involuntarily. The doctor of Jipmer prescribed glasses of minus two but failed to improve her sight with them. We were greatly puzzled and worried. Fortunately my daughter had been to the Divine Mother of Sri Aurobindo Ashram on her birthday. The Mother, after glancing at her, advised me to take Vijay Laxmi to Dr. Agarwal. "Who is Dr. Agarwal?" I enquired at the gate of the Ashram. A few days later my friend Bableshwar took us to the **SCHOOL FOR PERFECT EYESIGHT** to meet Dr. Agarwal. There were many patients waiting to meet the doctor. At the appointed time Dr. Agarwal carefully examined my daughter and after the examination he sat quietly. When I enquired whether there was any hope of improvement, the doctor called a boy-patient who had also been semi-blind about a month before, but now had perfect normal vision. "How can this be?" I doubted. Then I questioned the boy personally. It was a great relief to me when the boy narrated his story and the cure. Yet, I wanted to ascertain from the doctor the prospects for Vijay Laxmi. "Your daughter too will become all right, have patience and supply the materials I need for her treatment," the doctor said. We felt very happy and the next day I bought a set of colour pencils, a ballpen, a few notebooks, a ball, etc.

The sun was shining and the rays were very pleasant; the assistant applied **RESOLVENT** 200 to the eyes of Vijay Laxmi and, while facing the sun, she began to move her body, head and eyes from side to side like a pendulum. After a few minutes she washed the eyes with a pink lotion called **OPHTHALMO** and sat comfortably in the Palming-room. The doctor showed her how to do palming in the correct way. Then she played with a ball, did some drawing, swayed her body and read some letters of the chart. At times she was taken to the dark-room to concentrate on the candle flame. My daughter greatly enjoyed the treatment whenever she was called in the clinic. At home I had advised my wife not to scold her at any time but to help her in the treatment.

The results of this kind of treatment were wonderful. From the very first day my daughter's vision began to improve both for distance and near. She began to read smaller letters and finally she could easily read fine print with gentle blinking. By blinking the expression of the eyes and face changed.

Formerly she used to stare at objects and in this way had developed the habit of squinting. Now she reads her book well, and sees movies on Saturdays.

P. A. to The Governor, Pondicherry.

Myopia Cured Without Personal Assistance

The efficiency of the method of treating myopia and other visual defects by eye education is so great that I am constantly hearing of patients who have been able to improve their eyesight by the aid of information contained in my publications, without personal assistance. The writer of the following letter, a lady from Bombay, is a remarkable example of these cases:

"I acquired short sightedness in school, possibly due to improper way of seeing, posture and light and the power of glasses gradually increased to -3.0 in both eyes with years. After twelve years of living with glasses I found the spectacles most irksome. Then at the prompting of a friend I started practising eye exercises from Dr. Agarwal's book. This helped me to discard glasses totally within nine months. In my last visit to the Eye Doctor, he advised me to discard my glasses since my eyesight was normal. As I was prone to headaches without glasses I was wearing plane glasses for about three months but after that I learnt to live without glasses. I am forty years of age today and still enjoy normal vision."

Questions and Answers

Q: If reading is not the cause of myopia, then why do so many hard working students suffer from myopia ?

A: When the eye focuses itself at a near point as in reading, the condition is called accommodation. What happens in accommodation? The eye-ball is lengthened just like a camera when it focuses at a near point. When a student reads for long hours at a stretch, the eye is in a state of continuous accommodation and this condition is called excessive accommodation. After long study or, so to say, after excessive accommodation when the eye looks at distant objects, the vision is a little hazy, it takes some time for the eye to shorten its length so as to focus correctly and adopt the condition of rest. At this time if the eye makes an effort to see clearly, then the state of lengthening of the eye-ball continues and the eye becomes myopic. When this habit of straining becomes habitual, myopia sets in permanently. Some students escape because they do not continue to make an effort to see and are able to relax easily.

If after long study one can do palming and reading of the Snellen Test Card then the effect of the accommodation will pass away easily and quickly.

Q: In accommodation the eye-ball is lengthened, in myopia also the eye-ball is lengthened; then what is the difference between these two conditions?

A: Accommodation is without strain, without an effort to see, while myopia is due to an effort to see distant objects.

Q: If eye-strain is felt in reading, then what will happen?
A: The eye will become hypermetropic, there will be flattening of the eye-ball. It is why reading small print in dim light helps to counteract myopia.

Q: Why do eye specialists fail even to prevent myopia? My number has increased from -1.0 to -6.0.

A: It is because ophthalmic science regarding accommodation and errors of refraction is full of fallacies and falsehood. No attention is paid to minimise the strain to see distant objects and to relieve the mental strain which underlies the imperfect functioning of the eye. Further, a myopic patient sees well at a near point and reads better without glasses, but the doctor advises him to use glasses constantly.

Q: What will you advise then to a highly myopic patient?
A: Glasses may be used when necessary but not in reading. Palming may be done whenever convenient. Read the Snellen Eye Chart once a day without and with glasses, this will keep you aware about your eyesight. And read small print in dim light for a few minutes.

Q: How can I adjust myself in the class if I don't use glasses? I have to see the blackboard and read also.
A: Glasses may be used at that time but after the class do palming and avoid their use at home and at reading time.

Q: Why do you advise glasses for some and for some not?
A: Because some need their use, while others can manage without them and feel more relaxed.

Q: How is it that one eye becomes highly myopic while the other remains normal or little myopic?
A: Each eye functions separately; one may strain more than the other.

Q: What goes wrong in myopia and how can that defect be corrected?
A: (1) The eye-ball is elongated and is unable to focus

correctly. To correct this defect read in dim light for sufficient time.

(2) Central fixation is lost. This defect can be corrected by central fixation exercises or by the memory of a small letter.

Q: My vision is very poor even with glasses of -16 and I get temporary attacks of blindness. Gradually the vision is failing. Can your treatment help me?

A: I assure you that your eyes can be greatly benefited and you may come here for treatment.

Q: I am shortsighted and using glasses for five years. The number of glasses has not increased and I feel quite comfortable. The only difficulty is that sometime my eyes get tired after reading too much.

A: This is harmless myopia and you can continue with your glasses to see distant objects. While reading you should not use them because your reading sight is quite good without glasses. Do palming after reading. Read fine print.

Q: My one eye is myopic and the other hypermetropic. Since I have been using glasses, I have developed a dull headache, my memory is also affected. What do you advise?

A: As you can see well at a distance with one eye, and read well with the other, you should not use glasses. You don't need them at all.

One eye conveys a bigger image, while the other conveys a smaller image when the glasses are being used; and the mind has to fuse these different images and then it goes under a strain.

Q: I am myopic and I have to change my glasses quite frequently. Can you advise me something to check the increase of myopia?

A: (1)   Read without glasses.

          (2)   Read in dim light.

          (3)   Practise palming several times a day.

          (4)   Read the Snellen Eye Chart at ten feet without and with glasses, with gentle blinking.

Q: Why do you recommend to read in dim light? Everyone ridicules me when I study in dim light.

A: You are shortsighted. By reading in dim light for sufficient time hypermetropia is developed and hypermetropia neutralises the myopia. You can test this fact that by reading in dim light for sufficient time the distant vision is improved. While reading the distant chart you should blink at each letter. When reading in dim light is aided by central fixation, the improvement lasts longer.

Q: I sit in the verandah to practise on the eye chart to improve my distant vision. You have advised me to read in dim light and then to practise on the eye chart in good light. How to make such an arrangement?

A: Take a bed cover of dark colour, fold it, then use it as a cover over yourself, adjust the cover in such a way that there is quite dim light inside and it is little difficult to read at about 12 inches.

Q: I see something flying before my eyes; the doctor says, "floating specks", for which he has no cure.

A: Practise long swing and palming frequently and get the habit of blinking. Then the floating specks will fade away.

Remember two important points:
  (1) When floating specks appear, ignore them.
  (2) Do not test whether they are still there or not.

Q: Doctor, is your system of treatment an alternative, or a substitute or complementary to the orthodox system of treatment?

A: It is an alternative, a substitute as well as complementary depending upon the circumstances.

A person quite comfortable with his glasses, when likes to undergo this treatment, it becomes an alternative.

Usually in lower degrees of errors of refraction, we substitute it (the relaxation method) for glasses.

In cases of high myopia, it goes hand in hand with glasses. Glasses aid the vision in those cases and the relaxation methods check further deterioration.

Q: I see a white image of the black letter when I close my eyes. Is it a natural or physiological phenomenon?

A: This is called after-image. It is not a natural or physiological phenomenon. After-image is the sign of strain. When one looks at the letter with central fixation, after-image does not appear, black or real image appears.

CHAPTER VI

ASTIGMATISM

In all cases of astigmatism one meridian of the cornea is more convex or less convex than all the other meridians. The astigmatic eye is not able to focus the light from any object correctly.

School children are often nervous and when the nervousness is considerable, a large amount of astigmatism may be produced by a strain of the eyes and mind. When rest is secured the astigmatism in school children promptly disappears. Closing the eyes and palming, with the help of a nearly perfect memory of some letter or other object, secures a considerable amount of rest. The more perfect the memory the greater is the rest and relaxation. Rest of the eyes and mind is also obtained after the child has practised long swing or central fixation or seeing best where the eyes were looking.

It is very helpful to demonstrate to the patient that astigmatism is caused by a stare or strain and that rest or relaxation of the eyes will bring about a cure of astigmatism. The memory of familiar objects with the eyes closed is a great help in obtaining relaxation and lessening the amount of astigmatism. It often happens that patients of astigmatism find it difficult to obtain relaxation, because they try to see too much of any one object at once and try to see several letters of the chart at a time. The mere act of seeing one side of a letter at a time makes it easier to imagine the vision of each part of a letter.

One very successful method to improve the sight in astigmatic patients is to look at the white spaces in between the lines of print and imagine them whiter, first with eyes closed, then with eyes open. Imagine as if the bottoms of the letters are resting upon the upper part of the white spaces. When the sight is shifted on the white lines, the lines of letters appear to move in the opposite direction. Reading of fine print in good light and in candle light alternately proves very beneficial in the treatment of astigmatism.

Often patients tell us: "How can I remember black? It is impossible for me to remember black." One person tried to remember a small black dot and failed and a number of his friends tried and failed. When people try to see one dot of a colon blacker than the other and fail, the cause of failure is a strain. This strain is a mental strain. By an effort, sight, memory and imagination are lost. It is astonishing to know that the memory of imperfect sight is so difficult and that it requires considerable time and patience to help a patient realize the facts. Most people believe that to do wrong is easy and are very much surprised when someone tells them contrary and still more surprised when the facts are demonstrated.

When the largest letter of the Snellen Test Card is regarded, the blackness of it, the clearness of it, are so much better that people erroneously believe that the imagination of a large letter is much easier than the imagination of one half of the letter. When one half of the letter is covered, some people can imagine successfully that one half of a largest letter on the card is just as black, clear, and distinct as the same letter very much smaller. By continued practice the size of the letter can be reduced to a very small area.

Once a father brought his daughter for eye testing and her vision was found quite normal. The father said to the child: "Can you tell that the largest letter on the test card is blacker than the very small letters." The child intelligently declared that the large letter was not blacker or clearer than the smaller letters. The father then asked his daughter how she explained that she could see the small letters better than the large ones. She replied that the reason she saw small letters better than large ones was because there was not so much to see.

Having good eyesight the child could very readily produce a considerable amount of astigmatism by an effort of which she was conscious. She could also relieve the strain quickly and see a small letter at fifteen feet moving from side to side. The moment she tried to stop the movement of the letter, she felt discomfort and showed the symptoms of astigmatism.

Improve Your Sight

If you have imperfect sight and desire to obtain normal vision without glasses, I suggest that you keep in mind a few facts. In the first place the normal eye does not have normal sight all the time, so if you have relapses in the beginning do not be discouraged. First test your sight with each eye on the Snellen Test Card at ten or twenty feet, and see how clearly you read the fine print at ten inches. Then close your eyes and rest them by palming for about half an hour. Then open your eyes for a moment and again test your sight with both eyes at the same time.

Your vision should be temporarily improved if you have rested your eyes. If your vision is not improved it means that you have been remembering or imagining things imperfectly and under a strain. With the eyes closed and covered, at rest, with your mind at rest, you should not see anything at all — all should be black. If you see different colours, you are not resting your eyes but you are straining them.

When persons with normal sight do palming they observe perfect darkness before their eyes and they do not suffer from pain, discomfort, or headache or fatigue. When a person with imperfect sight closes the eyes and rests them successfully the eye becomes normal for the time being. When such a person looks at the distance and remembers some letter, some colour, or some object perfectly, the eyes are normal and the vision is perfect.

One of the quickest and most satisfactory way of improving the sight is with a perfect imagination. The white centres of the letters are imagined by the normal eye to be whiter than the margin of the card, while the eye with imperfect sight imagines the white centres of letters to be less white than the margin of the card. Persons with imperfect sight have been cured very quickly by encouraging them to imagine the letters in the same way as the normal eye imagines them.

When reading small print in a newspaper or in a book the normal eye is able to imagine the white spaces between the lines whiter than they really are. The whiter the spaces are imagined the blacker the letters appear and more distinct they become.

Persons with imperfect sight do not imagine the white spaces between the lines of fine print that they are endeavouring to read, to be as white as the margin of the page. Persons with imperfect sight cannot read fine print until they become able to imagine the white spaces whiter than they really are.

By central fixation is meant the ability to see best where you are looking. When one sees a small letter clearly or perfectly it can be demonstrated that while the whole letter is seen at one time, one sees or imagines one part best at a time. The normal eye, when it has normal vision, sees one letter of a line best or one part of a letter best at a time.

The more perfect the imagination, the more perfect is the

sight. It is interesting to realize that the truth about vision
in all its manifestations does not obey the laws of physiology,
the laws of optics, the laws of mathematics, and to try to
explain it in some plausible way is a waste of time.

Most people have an imagination that is good enough to
cure them if they would only use it. One can improve the
memory and imagination by alternately remembering a letter
with the eyes closed for a minute or longer and then opening
them and remembering the same letter for a fraction of a
second. After a patient has become able, under favourable
conditions, to imagine mental pictures as well with the eyes
open as with the eyes closed, his cure can be obtained in a
reasonable length of time. One patient, for example, could see
the large letter at ten feet but by the memory of a letter, alternately with his eyes closed and with his eyes open, obtained
almost normal vision in a few weeks.

Reading some small print or fine print in dim light for fifteen
or thirty minutes at a time greatly helps the myopic patients
to improve the sight for distance. For example, a boy could
read only five lines of the chart from twenty feet and his vision
was recorded 20/50. He was trying to improve the sight
by palming but failed to improve considerably. As he could
not very well remember some mental picture perfectly, his
improvement was poor. When he was advised to read fine print
in dim light for ten-fifteen minutes at a stretch and then glance
at the white centres of the chart letters at twenty feet his improvement was very quick. He could easily read the normal
line. By repeated practice the vision permanently improved.
It is because reading in dim light greatly helps to reduce
myopia.

It is very important that all patients who desire to be cured
of imperfect sight should discard glasses. Going without

glasses has at least one benefit; it acts as an incentive to the patient to practice the right methods in order to obtain good eyesight.

Fine Print

Many near-sighted patients can read fine print at less than ten inches from their eyes, easily, perfectly, and quickly by alternately regarding the Snellen Test Card at different distances, from three feet up to fifteen feet or further. The vision may be improved, at first temporarily, and later by repetition a permanent gain usually follows.

It is a valuable fact to know that when fine print is read perfectly the near-sightedness disappears during this period. The reading can be maintained at first only for a fraction of a second, and later more continuously.

Near-sighted patients and others, with the help of fine print, can usually demonstrate that staring at a small letter always lowers the vision and that the same holds true when regarding distant letters or objects.

With the help of fine print, the near-sighted patients can also demonstrate that one can remember perfectly only what has been seen perfectly: that one imagines perfectly only what is remembered perfectly: and that perfect sight is only a perfect imagination.

A great many people are very suspicious of the imagination and feel or believe that things imagined are never true. The more ignorant the patients, the less respect do they have for their imagination or the imagination of other people. It comes to them as a great shock, with a feeling of discomfort and annoyance, that the perfect imagination of a known letter improves the sight for unknown letters of the Snellen Test Card.

Seven Truths of Normal Sight

1. Normal Sight can always be demonstrated in the normal eye, but only under favorable conditions.

2. Central Fixation: The letter or part of the letter regarded is always seen best.

3. Shifting: The point regarded changes rapidly and continuously.

4. Swinging: When the shifting is slow, the letters appear to move from side to side, or in other directions with a pendulum-like motion.

5. Memory is perfect. The color and background of the letters or other objects seen, are remembered perfectly, instantaneously and continuously.

6. Imagination is good. One may even see the white part of letters whiter than it really is, while the black is not altered by distance, illumination, size, or form, of the letters.

7. Rest or relaxation of the eye and mind is perfect and can always be demonstrated.

When one of these seven fundamentals is perfect all are perfect.

Specimen of Diamond Type or Fine Print

CHAPTER XIII

MEMORY AS AN AID TO VISION

WHEN the mind is able to remember perfectly any phenomenon of the senses, it is always perfectly relaxed. The sight is normal, if the eyes are open, and when they are closed and covered so as to exclude all the light, one sees a perfectly black field —that is nothing at all. If you can remember the ticking of a watch, or an odor or a taste perfectly, your mind is perfectly at rest, and you will see a perfect black when your eyes are closed and covered. If your memory of a sensation of touch could be equal to the reality, you would see nothing but black when the light was excluded from your eyes. If you were to remember a bar of music perfectly when your eyes were closed and covered, you would see nothing but black. But in the case of any of these phenomena it is not easy to test the correctness of the memory, and the same is true of colors other than black. All other colors, including white, are altered by the amount of light to which they are exposed, and are seldom seen as perfectly as it is possible for the normal eye to see them. But when the sight is normal, black is just as black in a dim light as in a bright one. It is also just as black at the distance as at the near-point, while a small area is just as black as a large one, and, in fact, appears blacker. Black is, moreover, more readible

138

Photographic Type Reduction

Patients who can read photographic type reductions are instantly relieved of pain and discomfort when they do so, and those who cannot read such type may be benefited simply by looking at it.

It is a fact that one can read fine print perfectly with a perfect relaxation, with great relief to eye-strain, pain, fatigue and discomfort, not only of the eyes, but of all the nerves of the body.

Fine print, even when not read, but simply regarded, helps to improve distant vision, and the ability to read fine print helps all those suffering from Astigmatism, Hypermetropia, Presbyopia and other eye troubles.

Photographic Type Reduction

Patients who can read photographic type reductions are instantly relieved of pain and discomfort when they do so, and those who cannot read such type may be benefited simply by looking at it.

Good Eyesight

Preservation of good eyesight is almost impossible without eye education. Remember some fundamental principles of perfect eyesight.

1. Many blind people are curable.
2. All errors of refraction are functional, therefore curable.
3. All defective vision is due to strain in some form. You can demonstrate to your satisfaction that strain lowers the vision. When you stare, you strain. Look fixedly at one object for five seconds or longer. What happens? The object blurs and finally disappears. Also, your eyes are made uncomfortable by this experiment. When you rest your eyes for a few moments the vision is improved and the discomfort relieved.
4. Strain is relieved by relaxation.

To use your eyes correctly all day long, it is necessary that you:

I. Blink frequently. Staring is a strain and always lowers the vision.

II. Shift your glance constantly from one point to another, seeing the part regarded best and other parts not so clearly. That is, when you look at a chair, do not try to see the whole object at once; look first at the back of it, seeing that part best and other parts worse. Remember to blink as you quickly shift your glance from the back to the seat and legs seeing each part best, in turn. This is central fixation.

III. Your head and eyes are moving all day long. Imagine that stationary objects are moving in the direction opposite to the movement of your head and eyes. When you walk about the room or on the street, notice that the floor or pavement seems to come towards you, while objects on either side appear to move in the direction opposite to the movement of your body.

A Case of Astigmatism

Q: My son often gets headache while reading; the doctor has prescribed glasses of +0.25 to correct his astigmatism. I want to know what is astigmatism. Is it curable by your treatment?

A: The cornea of the eye is circular like a watch glass. It has two principal meridians — one horizontal and one vertical, each at a right angle to the other. When one meridian is flatter or more convex than the other, the eye develops astigmatism. Astigmatism is curable like other errors of refraction by eye education and mental relaxation exercises. Reading fine print is extremely helpful in such cases.

Q: What is mixed astigmatism. Is it also curable?

A: In mixed astigmatism one meridian is flatter than the normal, while the other meridian is more convex than the normal. The result is that the eye needs plus and minus lenses in the same eye. To make the subject interesting I give here the story of a patient — a report written by her father:

Report

My daughter Kavita is about 8 years old. I think it was her fifth birthday party, when she appeared before her tiny friends in a very serious mood, wearing an elderly look. She had not put on her grandma's specs, they were her own. How funny! How silly! and they were designed to be her life-long companion. No medical practitioner, no eye specialist grants divorce with spectacles, once you get along with them. There is only one person, an old inmate of Sri Aurobindo Ashram, who recommends such divorces. I shall tell you the story of my daughter.

At a young age, specially when she started her K. G., she had complained several times of headaches. Further, she was getting a cold and cough every two months. We took her first to an E.N.T. (Ear, Nose, Throat) Specialist. He found nothing wrong. We were also in touch with the Dentist. He had also nothing to say. Then we went to a well-known Eye Specialist of our Bangalore city. My daughter could hardly read the test chart half-way. The child of 5 was then taken to a dark room. The doctor went on saying, "See here, see there, see over my head, etc." Next day he tried several glasses, asking her, "This better or that? Now which is better?" and so on. The doctor managed to prescribe compound glasses with the following power:

R.E.   —1.5 sph.+3.0 cyl. axis 90
L.E.   —0.5 sph.+2.5 cyl. axis 90

We were puzzled to see the numbers where one axis is plus, the other minus. The doctor said that the eyes were very weak, and she could never think of getting rid of glasses. He asked us to go to him every year for a check-up.

So in October 1966, the doctor again examined my daughter's eyes and prescribed higher glasses:

R.E.   —2.0 sph.+4.0 cyl. axis 90
L.E.   —1.0 sph.+3.5 cyl. axis 90

Then one fine day we went to Pondicherry in connection with the school of Sri Aurobindo Ashram. We also took the opportunity to meet Dr. R. S. Agarwal, of whom we had heard sometime back. He examined my daughter's eyes very carefully and said her eyesight could become normal. He was confident in his words. Further, his elderly disposition and loving tone gave us full hope. He asked us to come one month in advance before the school opened at Pondicherry.

And thus we again came to Pondicherry about 3 weeks before the school re-opened. We went to Dr. Agarwal. He advised us to bring a set of colour pencils, one ruled note book, one blank note book, one dot pen, one pencil. Wonderful prescription! My daughter loved to have all that. Then daily in the morning we went to the doctor. My daughter could easily spend one and a half hour in his eye clinic. She was given a ball to play with. But all these were exercises for eyes. Playing with a ball gave her the correct way of blinking; like that all other things were important. Further, daily she was going to a dark-room, but with a candle burning. She was asked to read a small book with fine print in it. This too was interesting. The doctor used to make a group of 4-5 children and give them different games of eyesight to play in sequence. Every morning was a delightful morning.

Now I shall tell you the results. On the first day when we went to Dr. Agarwal, she was not able to read the last four lines on his chart from a particular distance without or with glasses. After 15 days of treatment she was able to read 3 further lines on his chart. What a wonderful result! Is it not like magic? My daughter was so happy when she learnt that no more spectacles would be needed in her whole life. And all these results were achieved in 15 days! Even when we go to a surgeon for any operation, he will take more than 15 days. And here her eyes were cured with a set of colour pencils, a note book and a candle!

K. C. Anand

Astigmatism Relieved by Eye Education

The belief about the incurability of Astigmatism is a dogma and a true scientist will always resist such a conservative idea. Dr. A. S. Drooby M.D., a well-known Psychiatrist of Lebanon, relates his experience to illustrate this fact:

"After only two days of Dr. Agarwal's treatment the present writer had a beneficial experience, in which astigmatism of many years standing was relieved. But before this is explained in greater detail, it would be worthwhile to relate the history of the case.

"As there is a great deal of printed matter to be read in this modern world, a system of reading called 'Fast or Rapid Reading' has been developed. The principles of fast reading are that one keeps the head stationary and moves the eyes only, also individual letters are not observed but one views whole words only. However the main process to achieve fast reading is to fixate the eyes upon the middle of the printed line (of a standard book size), and to shift the sight down the middle of the page, thus diminishing the eye movement to a minimum.

"Owing to bilateral astigmatism the present writer has worn glasses for the last 23 years, this astigmatism being combined with myopia of-1.5 in both eyes. The left eye was more affected than the right, with the net outcome that without glasses only the right eye would see or do the reading.

"The treatment at The School for Perfect Eyesight starts with the application of Resolvent 200 in the eyes, then sitting facing the sun with eyelids closed and rocking the body gently from side to side. This was followed by 5 minutes' palming, then the reading of fine print in bright, dim, and candle light.

"After only 2 days of treatment the writer had the following beneficial experience. Under the treatment one is advised during reading to move the head slightly with the movement of the eyes, and it was noted that by following this advice the print started to appear neater and darker.

"Another exercise consisted of reading through a hole of $1/_2$ inch diameter cut out of a card, this card is moved across the printed page so that one can only see a small length of the print at a time. By practising this exercise the print popped out as if enlarged from the hole, and there was no more blurring. For that moment the astigmatism was gone. Also reading with the left eye only and without the card, it was found that the print came out clearly and neatly.

"A comparison was then made between the new way of reading and the old, viz. reading with a movement of the head, and reading with the head fixed. Reading with head movement was found to be easier, and without blurring of the print. Reading without head movement brought back the astigmatic effect, and the sensation of eye-strain reappeared.

"This experience makes one take the orthodox optometrist's

management with a grain of salt. One also begins to question the wisdom of quickly correcting the refraction error with the use of lenses when a more natural and hygienic procedure is available. Furthermore a person applying the Agarwal method is given the chance, at least, (confirmed by others) to check the advance of myopia. With the use of lenses it is notorious that progressively higher dioptrics are required.

"The Bates-Agarwal technique is recommended whole-heartedly by this patient."

Questions and Answers

Q: I am a teacher. What instructions will you give so as to help the students?

A: 1. Perfection is the aim of our life. Under the modern conditions preservation of good eyesight is not possible without eye education. We recommend a plan of eye education for the schools.

2. **How to test the Sight?** Keep the eye chart at 20 feet distance and read it with each eye separately. Write the results in the form of a fraction. The numerator of the fraction is always the distance of the chart from the eyes. The denominator always denotes the number of the line of the chart read. If you can read the line marked 20 feet at twenty feet distance with the right eye, the vision is 20/20 (Normal); if you can read the line marked 50 feet at twenty feet distance with the left eye, the vision is 20/50 (Defective).

To test the near vision take the Fundamentals chart and hold it at 10 inches. Note which number you are able to read. The normal eye can read the smallest type of the Fundamentals.

3. The teacher, who holds the first period of the class, will see that the students, after palming, read the eye chart from

their seats silently, first with both eyes, then with each eye separately, avoiding any pressure on the eye-ball. Reading of the same familiar eye chart with gentle blinking is a wonderful eye education. Every home and every class should have the eye chart. Splendid results will be obtained if each teacher, before he holds the class, tells the students to do **Palming.**

4. **What is Palming?** Close the eyes and cover them with the palms of the hands avoiding any pressure on the eye-balls. Keep the eyes covered for about five minutes and imagine something interesting and familiar.

5. **How To Read?** Hold the book within twelve inches. Blink gently at each line. Do not be in a hurry to finish the book. Reading very fast usually causes strain in the eyes and mind. Reading small print and reading at a close distance is good for the eyes.

6. Reading under bright electric light is harmful because the light reflected from the paper causes strain to the eyes. Light just sufficient to read is good for them.

7. For quick relief of pain in the eye-balls and headache, reading fine print under candle light usually acts as a miracle. Get the habit of reading fine print daily and you will be saved from all eye troubles of old age.

8. Staring is bad. Tell the students to blink gently and frequently while seeing objects, reading books or watching the cinema. In wrong blinking the upper lid touches the lower lid with a jerk.

9. Students who find it difficult to get rid of eye strain or headache or defective vision may be sent to the School for Perfect Eyesight.

Q: When I go out in the sun I often get a headache. Can I use dark glasses or goggles?

A: If you have a liking for sun-glasses, you may use mild-coloured ones, but usually all such glasses make the eyes more sensitive and unhealthy.

When you go out in the sun, keep the lids lowered and blink frequently; then there will be natural protection from light and heat; imagine that the side objects and the road are moving backwards as one has the impression while travelling in a train — poles and trees appearing to rush past in the opposite direction. This also lessens the strain.

Every morning take a little sun-treatment. Face the sun with eyes closed for a few minutes. This will strengthen your eyes.

Q: What is Snellen Test Card or Eye Chart?

A: The Snellen Eye Chart has letters printed in varying sizes. It is used to test the eyesight for distance. The smallest letter seen on the eye chart from 10 feet or 20 feet is a measure of your distance vision.

It is a very useful thing for eye education so as to prevent and cure defective eyesight for distance.

Q: I suffer from hypermetropic astigmatism and feel quite comfortable with glasses. Do you advise me to go under your treatment?

A: Better continue the use of glasses till you feel any discomfort or deterioration in eyesight.

Q: I use glasses of -6 but I do not use them at the time of physical exercises. What causes pain in my eyes while doing physical exercises and how to cure it?

A: You are straining your eyes. Keep the lids a little lowered while doing any physical exercise and blink often.

Q: What was the trouble with Krishna Roy, a friend of mine? She was "blind" in her left eye and now she sees quite normally with that eye. How did she get cured in your clinic?

A: She had been having Amblyopia in her left eye since childhood. The word Amblyopia means blindness, the eye cannot be helped by glasses and for this no apparent or sufficient cause can be found in the constitution of the eye. She was cured by eye education and mental relaxation exercises.

Q: Previously I had the notion that reading under a bright light was good for my eyes. But now I find that reading in semi-darkness is helpful and avoids strain. Previously 20 minutes reading used to tire my eyes, now two hours reading produces no strain. Can you explain this fact?

A: In bright light the glare reflected from the paper creates strain in the eyes.

Q: Why do you advise to read the same Snellen Test Card daily as a means of eye education? Children have learnt it by heart.

A: You cannot see anything perfectly unless you have seen it before. When the eye looks at an unfamiliar object it always strains more or less to see that object, and an error of refraction is always produced. When the eyes regard a familiar object, however, the effect is quite otherwise.

This is why I recommend reading the same familiar Snellen Test Card.

Q: My father often tells me to stop seeing the cinema. Is the cinema really harmful for the eyes?

A: Cinematograph pictures can be made a means of improving the eyes. When they hurt the eyes, it is because the person strains to see them. If this tendency to strain can be overcome by gentle blinking, the vision is always improved and if the practice of viewing pictures is continued, many eye troubles are relieved.

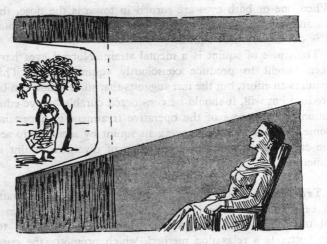

Correct way of watching a film

Chapter VII

Squint and Amblyopia

When one or both eyes are turned in towards the nose, the condition is called convergent squint. When the eyes turn out, it is called divergent squint.

The cause of squint is a mental strain. Normal eyes have been taught to produce consciously squint at will. This requires an effort, but the fact suggests that since squint can be produced at will, it should be considered curable by eye education. The success of the operative treatment is uncertain. Some children produce convergent squint by straining to see the end of the nose. The production of divergent squint is difficult.

Treatment: Since squint is caused by an effort or strain to see, mental relaxation is the fundamental part of the successful treatment. This may explain why teaching the eyes to see better is a relaxation method, which promotes the cure of the squint. When the vision is improved of each eye to normal, the eyes become straight. If somehow the relaxation treatment fails to correct the squint, then only one may think of the operation.

Young children are cured of squint by swinging the whole body in a circular direction and swinging them strongly enough to lift their feet from the floor. While swinging the hands of the child are held by the hands of an adult who may be swinging him. At the same time the child is encouraged to look upwards as much as possible. The little patient will immensely enjoy this form of exercise. Games of all kinds have been practised with much benefit to the squint in children.

When double vision appears with squint, it is very annoying. Any method, which secures relaxation, corrects the double vision and lessens the squint. Many patients are greatly benefited by palming, long swing and reading fine print in good light and candle light. Undoubtedly blinking is a great aid to cure the squint as well as double vision. When this is not sufficient, one may select the exercise of memory or imagination.

The Snellen Test Card may be useful in the cure of squint. While swaying from side to side, standing a few feet from the card, all stationary objects in the field of vision may appear to be moving in the opposite direction to the sway. While practising the sway, the whiteness of the card improves while the blackness of the letters becomes darker and the vision improves. If one eye is normal and the other defective, the good eye is covered for several hours a day, so that bad eye may learn functioning in the right way.

Recently two teachers of the Centre of Education developed a squint in their right eye due to working on the microscope with a strain. When the squint appeared, double vision followed and this was very disturbing and annoying. They were cured by palming, long swing and reading fine print or photographic type reduction with gentle blinking. Frequent palming kept their eyes under relaxation. In such cases football swing is also very helpful.

What is footfall swing? Take a tennis ball and move it with your foot, the sight moves with the ball but the floor appears to move backward. This imagination of the floor moving backward brings good relaxation. After playing this game for a few minutes one may read fine print or the Snellen Test Card at varying distances.

Usually there is a lowering of vision in the squinting eye which cannot be improved by glasses, and this condition is called *amblyopia* which is supposed to be incurable, but by relaxation methods of eye education, amblyopia is cured quite rapidly in many cases.

Double Vision

Many children and adults suffer from double vision which is often very annoying. One of the best methods for double vision is palming for longer or shorter periods of time. Any method of treatment which brings relaxation, corrects the double vision.

Some patients are benefited by standing with the feet about one foot apart, the arms and hands hanging loosely at the sides, while they sway the body slowly, continuously, easily, from side to side. The swaying of the body from side to side lessens or prevents concentration or other efforts to see. Should this not be sufficient to cure double vision, one may practise blinking, central fixation on the Snellen Test Card with frequent palming.

While swaying before the Snellen Test Card from side to side, the letters on the chart appear to move in the opposite direction. When the sway is short and slow the whiteness of the letters improves, while the blackness of the letters becomes darker and the double vision disappears.

If the trouble is in reading, move the sight on the white lines in between the lines of print without any effort to read and observe the lines of letters which appear to be moving in the opposite direction. When successful, the whiteness in the letters appears whiter while the blackness of the letters grows prominent. The vision is improved and double vision disappears.

The imagination of a small "O" while glancing at the

letters of the Snellen Test Card or while reading fine print is a great help in the cure of double vision.

A girl was suffering from squint and double vision. By frequent palming and practice on the Snellen Test Card with gentle blinking all the time, she was completely cured.

A Student's Palming Composition

1. Palming has greatly helped me to relax my nerves of the head and eyes and of the whole body. I often suffered from headache in the midst of my work and at times had vomiting. The whole body was under strain. But now everything has become easy and I no more suffer from headache.

2. One day my brother had severe headache. He was wearing glasses. I told him to start palming. After half an hour the vision considerably improved. He teaches others how to do palming to obtain relaxation.

3. Palming and reading of the Snellen Test Card daily has enabled me to preserve good eyesight. It gives me strength in my imagination, and I can do my work much better.

4. I told my mother to do palming, I said it would help her, but she did not believe me. One day I said, "Mother, palm." She said, "All right." Finally a week later she could see clearly and began to read fine print. She said, "I am glad I did what you told me."

5. We have a palming lesson every day. While we are palming we have a little music in order to think of something pleasant. It has cured many weak-eyesight students and relieved their pains of the head. It is spreading everywhere, and we see lots of people doing it now.

6. Palming is a wonderful treatment for the eyes and mind. I do not get excited now and my eyesight has become normal.

I get good sleep. My sister is cured of her squint.

Blindness or Amblyopia

When the normal eye has normal sight, it is constantly moving. When it has imperfect sight or is partially or completely blind, it is always seeing stationary objects or letters stationary, or is making an effort to do so. These two truths suggest the prevention or cure of blindness. When adults, school children and others are taught to imagine stationary objects to be always moving, the vision always improves.

When the sight is poor and cannot be improved promptly by glasses, the cause usually is due to amblyopia. The word amblyopia means blindness. In amblyopia the vision is less in the region or the centre of sight, hence central fixation is always found to be quite defective.

Since it is a truth that staring, concentration, causes imperfect sight, any treatment which relieves strain should always improve the sight or improve the vision in amblyopic cases. Recently I treated five children of the Centre of Education who were suffering from amblyopia. Apparently the eyes looked quite all right but the vision was poor both for distance and reading and could not be improved by glasses. When they looked at the chart letters, heir eyes were stationary, there was no blinking, there was no movement of the eye-balls. All these children gained normal vision by palming, swinging and candle practice. They were taught blinking and how to move the eyes with the movement of the head by means of a ball. They moved the ball from one hand to the other and shifted the sight with the movement of the ball.

The great mistake that has been commited for the last one hundred years or more is in ignoring amblyopia. Most doctors believe amblyopia incurable. Time after time patients with amblyopia have been treated in my clinic with success by relaxation methods.

In the case of young children methods have to be modified. There are many ways in which this can be done, and it is important to devise a variety of means so that the child will not weary of them. For the same reason the presence of other children is at times desirable. There must be no compulsion and no harshness, for as soon as any method ceases to be pleasant it ceases to be beneficial.

The needle, the brush, the pencil, kindergarten and Montessori material, picture books, playing cards, etc., may all be utilised for purposes of eye training. If one eye is normal, the other amblyopic, then the good eye is to be covered and the bad eye is trained on such material. At first it will be necessary to use rather large objects and forms, but as the sight improves, the size must be reduced. A child may begin to sew, for instance, with a coarse needle and thread, and will naturally take large stitches. As its sight improves a finer needle should be provided, and the stitches will naturally be smaller.

One very amusing practice for children is to sit on a small stool with a chart placed at five feet or farther. The child then runs around the stool while bouncing the ball. After every five rounds he sits down, closes the eyes and then reads the chart letters while blinking on each letter.

Many interesting games can be devised with playing cards. "Slap Jack" is a good one, as it awakens intense interest and great quickness of vision is required to slap the Jack with the hand the moment its face appears on the table.

These ideas are only suggestions, and any intelligent parent will be able to add to them.

Suggestions

1. Imagine Things are Moving All The Time

When riding in a railroad train, when one looks out of the car window, telegraph poles and other objects, although they are stationary, appear to be moving. To stop the movement is impossible, and the effort to do so may be very uncomfortable. The greater the effort, the greater the discomfort, and is the cause of heart sickness, headaches and nausea. It can be demonstrated that any movement of the head and eyes produces an apparent movement of stationary objects.

2. Blink Often

By blinking is meant to make short and rapid movements of the eyelids. When done properly, things are seen continuously and they always move with a quick jump in various directions. Regarding stationary objects without blinking is an effort, a strain which always lowers the vision.

3. Read The Snellen Test Card Daily

School children and others are often cured of imperfect sight by reading a familiar card at ten or fifteen feet distance, first with both eyes and then with each eye separately. It is the only method practised which prevents MYOPIA in school children.

4. Fine Print

Read fine print at six inches or nine inches when possible every night and morning. If not possible, do the best you can. Just regarding the white spaces between the lines of fine print without reading the letters is a benefit.

5. Palming
Palm for five minutes several times a day.

Permanent Improvement

Many patients find that while it is easy for them to obtain a temporary improvement in their sight by palming a sufficient length of time or by other methods, they do not seem to hold it permanently. In this connection it is well to remember that the normal eye with normal sight can only maintain normal sight permanently by consciously or unconsciously practising the slow, short, easy swing. When the normal eye has imperfect sight it can always be demonstrated that the swing stops from an effort. When the normal eye has normal sight, the eyes are at rest and all the nerves of the body feel comfortable. When the swing stops, one always feels more or less uncomfortable. Perfect sight can only be obtained easily, without effort. To have imperfect sight always requires a strain or an effort which stops the swing. Near-sighted patients who have normal vision for reading at the near point become able, when their attention is called to it, to demonstrate that they are more comfortable when reading the fine print than they are when they fail to see distant objects clearly.

Persons with imperfect sight should imitate the eye with normal sight by practising a perfect memory, a perfect imagination, a perfect swing, without effort, with perfect comfort all the time that they are awake. Reading of fine print daily in good light and in candle light is a wonderful help to prevent and cure defective eyesight. To obtain a permanent cure it is necessary that children should devote a few minutes a day to palming, swinging, and reading the Snellen Test Card as long as they attend school.

Eye Strain During Sleep

Many people complain that when they first wake up in the morning, they are tired, that they have headaches, and that their eyesight is bad. Later on in the day their eyes feel better, and the vision becomes all right.

Many persons strain much more in their sleep than they ever do when they are awake. They see all sorts of unfamiliar dreams, some even scream while in sleep. Of course, people when unconscious of their acts during sleep, are not aware of their dreams or eye-strain.

Eye-strain during sleep is sometimes difficult to treat. Some cases are benefited by palming for about half an hour before retiring. Others, by practising the long swing before and after sleep, have found great relief. Some persons are benefited by shortening their hours of sleep with the help of an alarm clock. One patient had the alarm set for 3 a.m. He would then get up from bed and practise the long swing and palming with the result that he slept the rest of the night very comfortably, and awoke the next morning with little or no evidence of eye-strain during sleep.

Some people are able to get good sleep by doing moderate muscular or breathing exercises. A girl patient was cured by reciting a prayer or a devotional song many times before going to bed. A boy was advised to run around a chair before and after sleep and this had a very good effect in curing his eye-strain during sleep.

How My Blind Eye Got Cured

When I was twelve, I often suffered from headaches and my eyes were examined. It was found that my left eye had always been blind, I could not see even the biggest letter of the eye chart and no glasses could improve the vision of this eye.

At the end of May 1967 Dr. Thadani came to our School for the eye checkup. All the students were excited to see whose eyes were best. They read the Snellen Test Card perfectly — all except me. I knew about my bad eye but the children were stunned to see that I could hardly read even the big letter from 20 feet with my left eye though the right eye was quite normal. Dr. Thadani gave a long discourse on how to improve my eyesight with natural methods. He said that since I had only one good eye, if something happened to it, then I would be quite blind. Would I like it? He encouraged me to go to Dr. Agarwal's Eye Clinic and be under his treatment. He talked to me about his own eyes and how at the age of 69 he still read without glasses. So finally I decided to go to Dr. Agarwal.

It was on the 4th June 1967, Sunday, that I went to his clinic. There I saw many patients, mostly children; they were busy doing their eye exercises. The doctor welcomed me very warmly. He tested my eyes carefully and examined them in the dark room. Immediately he told me what was wrong with my left eye. He explained to me that I had Amblyopia, which means blindness: the eye cannot be helped with glasses, and for this no apparent or sufficient cause can be found in the constitution of the eye.

At first I was given a book *Better Sight*, then *Mind and Vision* to read. I learnt many things about the eye and I found the books quite interesting. I was surprised at myself, for usually I am not in the least interested in medical subjects; I just don't have the nerve to read all that with quaint names. But luckily the books were quite simple and I was glad to read them.

On the very first day Dr. Agarwal told me with confidence that I would be cured in two months' time. I was overjoyed and agreed to take up his treatment as guided. I somehow just wanted to be cured. And surprisingly within two months, with regular exercises for about two hours a day, my sight slowly came back, then considerably improved and I began to read fine print. I also saw the cinema on every Saturday with the left eye only and I greatly enjoyed it.

I was much obliged and happy at the time and energy and interest the doctor alloted to me, so I gave up many other activities which were very dear to me, for nothing could be dearer than to be healthy and strong and free of all artificial contraptions. To get back one's sight is to see the world with a new light and new vision.

One day without the doctor's permission I was doing some fret-work at home. I was feeling the strain in my eyes but I continued the work. Suddenly severe headache developed, I could not sleep on that night. Next morning I came to the doctor very much depressed and told him all about my headache. He gave me something to smell and asked me to do palming till the headache was relieved. After half an hour I was quite relaxed.

Such a love of the doctor for his patient I had never realized before. Along with the improvement of eyesight my inner being also began to develop by his touch and influence. My patience, forbearance, concentration power considerably increased and I felt more self-confident and strong within.

A Teacher

A Case of Hysterical Amblyopia

I was upset when a report was received from Sri Aurobindo International Centre of Education that my daughter Ange had developed very bad eyesight, she could not see the blackboard letters and often made mistakes in copying from her books. This was an indication that her eyesight was bad both for far and near. Next day I made an appointment with Dr. Agarwal and brought Ange to his eye clinic. When her eyesight was tested, Ange could see only the top letter from ten feet distance and her vision was recorded 10/200, and at the near point she could see about quarter inch size letters. But then when I showed paintings and drawings of Ange to the doctor, then he remarked that Ange was suffering from Hysterical Amblyopia.

What is Amblyopia? The doctor said, "The word Amblyopia means blindness without any apparent cause. The patient does not know what is wrong; neither does the doctor, yet the patient cannot see. Under certain conditions of mental strain Ange failed to see while under other favourable conditions she could see very well."

Dr. Agarwal put some questions to me and found out the cause of mental strain which produced temporary blindness or loss of eyesight. Often the teacher at the school or the father at home scolded Ange and forced her to adopt a certain discipline and learn Arithmetic for which she has absolutely no liking. The doctor told me that unless this tension was relieved at home and school, the treatment would not produce good results. The matter was placed before the Divine Mother by Mr. Kireet. Since then Ange has found that the teacher and the father treated her very kindly and did not force any discipline. Yet Ange is a very sensitive girl, she expresses herself freely and joyfully in a disciplined way. She has the energy to learn many things.

Further Dr. Agarwal stated that some children when they enter the schoolroom, become nervous especially when the teacher is harsh and unkind or when the child has to study subjects for which there is no interest or liking. This nervousness causes mental strain, and when there is mental strain, the eyes also feel strain and the result is loss of sight. It is because vision is greatly associated with the mind. What we see is the mind's interpretation of the retinal images, in other words, the vision is mostly our imagination. By the improvement of imagination the causes of eye trouble are relieved and the sight is improved.

On the day of treatment I brought 2 red balls, a set of coloured pencils, drawing books and some sweets. At first we played with the balls, the doctor and the assistant also joined the game which was organised by Ange herself. When the game and its fun was over, Ange traced a drawing and coloured it. At times she did palming on the rocking chair. A Snellen Test Card was placed at about fifteen feet distance from Ange. The doctor asked Ange to read the chart letters and write them around the drawing in different colours. It was a great surprise to all of us when Ange read the last line of the chart and wrote it correctly on her drawing. Her vision was recorded more than normal, that is, 15/10. On the next turn she read fine print quite easily. At home she daily read the chart from ten feet distance. All the symptoms of temporary blindness were chased away by this simple treatment.

It is a truth that when children are in motion, they feel greatly relaxed. For that running, dancing, playing, rocking, reading while shifting the sight from side to side, etc., are all very helpful.

Each day at the School for Perfect Eyesight was a very joyful day for Ange. And today we all feel very happy to see Ange enjoying good eyesight and this short note is an expression of our gratitude.   Ruth

Cure of Squint

An old teacher of our Centre of Education was maintaining good eyesight with her bifocal glasses. Suddenly one day, she felt that she was seeing double images of the object. She observed that her left eye had almost gone blind; it could see neither at a distance nor at near and her vision was very hazy with or without glasses. When she looked into the mirror it greatly shocked and depressed her to see that convergent squint had developed in her left eye and it was quite prominent.

On examination in the dark room it was found that the inside of the eye was quite normal. We assured the patient that her sight will be all right within a few weeks and she began to follow the treatment:

1. Keep the eyes closed and move the body gently from side to side and not to open the eyes widely at any time and stop reading and writing completely. In the breakfast she was advised to take only fruits and a cup of tea. Egg, butter, bread which made up for her usual breakfast were completely stopped. This relieved the tension and she found her mind and body quite relaxed. By following this first instruction for about a month, double vision almost disappeared and there was clarity in the vision. She felt the eyes and mind relaxed.

2. After a month she used to come daily for her treatment in the clinic for taking sun treatment, doing palming, long swing and candle practice. She had developed the good habit of blinking which is imperative in bringing about gratifying improvement in such cases, and in a month's time her left eye gained almost normal vision with a lower power of glasses; but this did not help in correcting her squint.

3. The constant presence of squint was due to some tension

and weakness of the muscle. It was not due to the paralysis of the external rectus muscle as it is generally believed. In such cases a special treatment 'Tarpana' helps very much to strengthen the weak muscle and correct the squint. The first course of treatment relieved the squinting state of the eyes temporarily. Squint was disappearing and reappearing. But after the third course of treatment which was after a fortnight, her convergent squint completely disappeared for good and the eye became normal both in appearance and function.

Another exercise which helped her to regain her lost binocular vision was daily practice on Amblyoscope. In the first days of her treatment she found it very difficult to fuse the images. Gradually, as the tension became less and the muscle became stronger the faculty of fusion developed. This was also helped by closing the good eye at home and doing all the household work for an hour or so with the bad eye (her squinting eye) only. Naturally, the bad eye learned to function without effort and strain. The use of the bad eye made the muscle stronger and in due course of time she could move her left eye outwards without having to move her head which was not at all possible when she came first.

The cause of such a sudden onset is a severe mental strain and the long standing habit of using the eyes improperly. It was worthwhile cross-questioning this teacher; for, towards the end the cause became crystal clear which by itself was a very great suggestive of treatment. It was found that her mind was burdened with anxieties and worries and that she used to feel spent up after a little work. Many other minor points such as these, helped us greatly in determining her treatment. Now that she is absolutely normal and that she has resumed her work she feels happy and grateful; greater is our pleasure to see her well and free of such a displeasing abnor-

mality which otherwise would have tinted her life with a shade
of unhappiness.

Furthermore, operations in such cases do not prove beneficial. On the contrary they may damage the functioning of the
eye. Operations can only correct the existing abnormality
temporarily but cannot relieve the root cause, namely-strain
upon the nerves responsible for the sound action of the
external rectus muscle.

Questions and Answers

*Q: My daughter is four years old, she has developed a squint
and her right eye turns towards the nose.*

A: Young children can usually be cured of squint by the
use of atropine. A one-percent solution is dropped into the
better eye or both eyes daily for about one year. The atropine
makes it more difficult for the child to see, and makes the sunlight disagreeable. In order to overcome this difficulty the
child has to relax the eye muscles, and the relaxation cures
the squint. Swaying the child in a circle is also very useful.

*Q: I use glasses for reading and am fifty years old. Without
glasses I cannot work. Now these glasses do not give clear vision.
What to do?*

A: Concentrate on a candle flame while counting one
hundred respirations. Read small print with glasses in good
light and in candle light.

*Q: I discarded glasses and I ride frequently on a cycle; I often
go on a trip in the car and after every trip I find my eyes stronger.
This, I think, is due to the rapid changing of focus in viewing
scenery going by so fast.*

A: The rapid motion compels rapid shifting and helps in relieving the strain.

Q: Every year I get inflammation in my eyes, the glare troubles me and I use dark glasses. Can my eyes be benefited?

A: Take sun treatment for a few minutes daily. At night practise concentration on a candle flame and read fine print.

Q: When I travel in a bus, my eyes are greatly strained.

A: Imagine side objects moving backwards, do not stare at any object. Better look at the movements of the conductor or read something so as to avoid the habit of staring.

Q: What is most helpful when one is highly myopic and finds it almost impossible to see without glasses?

A: Practise palming frequently and read fine print with gentle blinking in dim light.

Q: Why is fine print beneficial?

A: Fine print is beneficial because it cannot be read by a strain or effort, the eyes must be relaxed.

Q: How can I correct the vision of my three year old son, who won't palm and does not understand it? He is far-sighted.

A: Make a test card with black letters on white paper. The letters are to be composed of Es pointing in various directions. These Es are to be graduated in size, from about $3\frac{1}{2}$ inches to a quarter of an inch. Let the child read them from 10 to 20 feet away. Have him blink constantly while telling in which direction the Es are pointing.

Q: I have improved my sight by palming, but when I read for any length of time, the pain returns.

A: When you read and your eyes pain you, it means that you are straining your eyes. More frequent palming and reading fine print with gentle blinking will help you.

Q: Is it all right to palm while lying down? Is it better to sit or stand while doing so? If the arms get tired is it all right to rest the elbows on a desk or something like that while palming? Or is it best to hold the elbows up free from all support?

A: It is all right to palm while lying down. Palming should not be done while one is standing. The elbows should rest on a desk or on a cushion placed in the lap. One should be in as comfortable a position as possible while palming, in order to obtain the most benefit.

Q: If type can be seen more distinctly with the eyes partly closed, is it advisable to read that way?

A: No, it is not advisable to read that way because it is a strain, and alters the shape of the eye-ball.

CHAPTER VIII

EYE TROUBLES IN OLD AGE

Presbyopia

Presbyopia is the name given to the loss of power to use the eyes at the near point without the aid of glasses, which usually occurs after the age of forty. It is a noteworthy fact that many other eye troubles such as cataract, glaucoma and inflammation of the interior of the eye-ball start about this time. There are cases, however, in which the vision remains quite normal in both eyes long after the presbyopic age.

A man of sixty-five had quite good vision both for far and near. His vision on the Snellen Test Card was 20/10, and he could read the fine print at twelve inches. In reply to a query as to how he could possess normal vision at this age, he said that when he was about forty he began to experience difficulty in reading. He consulted an optician who advised glasses. He could not believe, however, that the glasses were necessary, because at times he could read perfectly without them. The matter interested him so much that he began to observe facts, a thing that people seldom do. He noted, first, that when he tried hard to see either at the near-point or at the distance, his vision invariably became worse, and the harder he tried the worse it became. Evidently something was wrong with this method of using the eyes. Then he tried to look at things without effort, without trying to see them. He also tried resting his eyes by closing them for five minutes or longer, or by looking away from the page that he wished to read, or the distant objects he wished to see. These practices always improved his sight and by keeping them up he not only regained normal vision but retained it for twenty-five years.

The fact is that presbyopia is due to strain. Glasses may enable the patient to read but cannot relieve the strain which underlies the imperfect functioning of the eyes. It is a matter of common experience that the vision declines rapidly after the patient begins to wear glasses. When people put on glasses because they cannot read fine print they often find that in a couple of weeks they cannot, without them, read the coarse print which was perfectly clear to them before. In some cases the decline of eyesight is quite fast and the oculist is compelled to change the glasses quite frequently, increasing the number each time.

Presbyopia is cured just as any other error of refraction is cured, by rest and relaxation. Some presbyopic patients are cured very quickly, others are very slow, but as a rule every one is benefited. When the improvement is very slow, glasses are permitted along with a few minutes exercise. Such patients are advised to concentrate on a candle flame and read fine print with glasses.

Central fixation on OM chart, shifting the sight on white lines, concentration on a candle flame, frequent palming, reading of fine print are very helpful to presbyopic patients.

While it is sometimes very difficult to cure presbyopia, it is fortunately easy to reduce the power of glasses or to prevent it. Persons who are approaching the presbyopic age, should start reading fine print in good light and in candle light alternately, bringing the print closer and closer to the eyes till it can be read at six inches. Thus you will escape, not only the necessity of glasses for reading, but all other eye troubles which so often darken the later years of life.

It is usually quite comfortable to use correct glasses for reading but the tendency of many doctors is to give a little higher number and that creates deterioration in eyesight quite fast. If such patients are advised to read fine print daily with glasses, they will be saved from many discomforts and eye troubles.

Patients who have myopia sometimes obtain normal vision just by removing glasses and not wearing them again for reading. Presbyopic patients have a tendency to read in bright electric light, and if the bright light reflects glare from the paper, then it causes harm and weakens the eyes. The light should be so arranged that there is no reflection from the paper. However, reading in candle light is immensely beneficial.

A Case of Presbyopia

It is a general belief that presbyopia or old age sight is a normal result of growing old, so at the age of forty-two when I experienced difficulty in reading, the natural impulse in me was to consult an eye specialist and get glasses. Since then I have been using glasses and at the age of sixty-four the number of my glasses was plus 3.5. Though I knew Dr. Agarwal very well, it never occurred to me that I could do away with glasses. I had taken the doctor's advice as a verdict that nothing else could replace glasses.

For sometime I was feeling heaviness or headache or strain in the eyes specially after reading and a sort of veil appeared before the eyes which made the vision defective. This trouble acted as a source of inspiration to consult our friend Dr. Agarwal whose wonderful cures we sometimes read of in *Mother India*.

About a week back one morning I happened to be in his eye clinic at the School for Perfect Eyesight. My glasses and vision were checked.

"Will you like to discard your glasses and get new vision?" he asked.

"It will be a blessing, but will it really be possible to discard glasses at this age?" I counter questioned.

"Leave these glasses with me for a week and undergo a short course of eye education and see the result," he advised.

Very gladly I consented to his advice and started the treatment. To my surprise the vision began to improve from the first sitting, and in a week's treatment I was able to read very small print easily. Now my near vision is as good as my distant vision. Dr. Agarwal has assured me that there will be no cataract or any other trouble if I could devote a few minutes daily to eye exercises. Though I keep a small number pair of glasses in my pocket, I hardly use them.

The process of treatment that I followed was first to apply *Resolvent* 200 and face the morning sun for a few minutes with the eyes closed, then after washing the eyes with eye lotion I practised *Palming*. When I closed the eyes and covered them with my palms I could see that it was all perfect dark before my eyes like black velvet. Then I looked at the candle flame while counting one hundred respirations. The next process was to shift the sight in between the lines of small print with gentle blinking and at frequent intervals I read the Snellen Chart placed in dim light at fifteen feet distance. This process enabled me little by little to read the small print. And when I could read the small print, the ordinary book print automatically became easy and legible. It was a surprise to me when the small print could be read easily. Then Dr. Agarwal explained everything.

A letter or a word is a combination of black and white. When you look at the white instead of concentrating on the black the eye muscles are relaxed and the eye is able to accommodate in a normal way. If people arriving at forty years of age adopt this simple process of reading some small print daily in good light as well as in candle light, they will be able to maintain good eyesight throughout their life and they will be saved from cataract and glaucoma and other eye troubles of old age. According to the view of Dr. Agarwal presbyopia is the result of strain, hence preventable and curable.

How is it fine print becomes clear after looking at some distant object? Answering this question Dr. Agarwal said that the strain at the distant object elongates the eye-ball so as to accommodate while reading. Such a practice is useful when one uses plus glasses.

An Inmate of the Ashram

Cataract

Cataract is a form of imperfect sight in which the lens of the eye becomes opaque. It usually begins after the age of fifty, and may progress in the course of a year or longer to complete blindness. But in some cases cataract develops very slowly; such a cataract is usually due to eye strain and can be greatly benefited by proper treatment.

If a nucleated eye-ball of an animal is squeezed with the aid of fingers, an opacity of the lens at once appears. When the squeeze is relieved, the lens at once becomes apparently perfectly clear.

There are two oblique and four straight or recti muscles on the outside of the eye-ball. The pressure of the two oblique muscles causes lengthening of the eye-ball while the four recti muscles shorten the eye-ball by their contraction. The pressure of the muscles can cause hardness of the eye-ball and formation of cataract also.

To obtain good vision, eye doctors remove the opaque lens by an operation. After the removal of the lens, the vision is materially improved by the use of strong glasses. But in many cases the good vision obtained after the operation does not remain good. In some cases without any apparent cause inflammation of the interior parts of the eye develops and is followed by serious loss of vision. All such cases can be greatly benefited if after the operation they can practise sun treatment and palming two or three times a day. They may read some small print also daily with their reading glasses. Such a treatment will prevent the loss of vision after the operation.

Cataract patients in the early stage can be cured partially or completely, especially when the development of cataract is slow, by eye education and mental relaxation. But if relaxation treatment fails to prevent and cure cataract we should consider this fact an evidence that strain is not the cause of the cataract.

TREATMENT. The vision of cataract patients improves by sun treatment and after palming, when the patient learns how to do it in the right way. Application of Resolvent 200 just before sun treatment helps in the treatment. But if the cataract has matured, it needs an operation.

Treatment which brings about relaxation in the eyes and mind has cured cataract after several months or longer. Among the many methods of treatment is a development of good memory and imagination. Practice of long swing and central fixation greatly helps when there is increased tension also.

When the patient is able to remember and imagine something perfectly, the vision is quickly improved, but if the same patient stares or makes an effort to see, the vision always becomes worse. This suggests a cure. But the great difficulty in many old persons is this that they find it difficult to relax sufficiently and they continue the habit of staring or straining the eyes. If they can learn the simple process of blinking and palming, they will find definite improvement.

Some cases of cataract acquire the ability to read fine print without glasses. When such patients are recommended to read fine print many times a day, the cataract becomes less and the vision improves. These cases are greatly benefited when they learn how to concentrate on a candle flame while counting one hundred respirations. The practice of reading fine print in good light and in candle light proves very helpful in the prevention and cure of cataract. Shifting the sight on white lines of fine print without any effort to read is a quick method to improve the sight in early cataract patients.

Questions and Answers

Q: What is cataract?

A: Cataract is an opacity of the lens in the pupil, which interferes with good vision. In many cases the spasm of external eye muscles is the cause of cataract and such cases are benefited by relaxation treatment.

Q: I have not seen with the right eye for one year. Doctors diagnose 'Cataract' and advise an operation. Can your treatment help me?

A: Operation is the right treatment when the cataract is matured.

Q: Is cataract curable in the early stage?

A: Cataract which is due to strain is curable and the vision is always improved by long palming and by concentration on candle flame.

Q: My both eyes have been operated upon for cataract and I use glasses but for sometime the vision has been gradually deteriorating.

A: Sun treatment and palming and reading small print with glasses will be very helpful to stop deterioration.

Q: What is the best preventive for cataract?

A: Apply *Resolvent* 200.

Concentrate on a candle flame.

Read small print.

Q: My right eye is quite all right but in the left a cataract is slowly developing.

A: Better arrest the growth of the cataract by the application of Resolvent 200 and relaxation treatment.

Q: My early cataract has been cured by your treatment but my eyes are irritated sometimes by the application of Resolvent 200.

A: Stop Resolvent 200 but continue the rest of the treatment.

Q: You have advised me operation for my cataractous eye; I thought you would cure it without an operation.

A: I advise according to the necessity.

Q: I have high myopia and a cataract is developing very slowly. Can I be benefited?

A: Apply Resolvent 200 and read fine print daily.

Q: Doctors diagnose glaucoma and cataract in my eyes but don't suggest anything to prevent blindness. Can I come to your clinic for treatment?

A: Yes, your eyes will be greatly benefited.

Q: *Is a great amount of floating specks an indication of cataract? When I am tired, these look like a swarm of bees crossing my eye-balls.*

A: No. Your particular strain produces floating specks. A different strain produces cataract. By relaxation both can be benefited.

Q: *If cataract is caused by some physical ailment, will your methods help?*

A: Yes, relaxation is always a benefit, not only to the eyes, but to all the nerves of the body.

Q: *My son has had cataract in both eyes since birth. What do you advise?*

A: If he is almost blind, then better get him operated upon.

Q: *What is the Mother's attitude to your eye treatment?*

A: The Mother wrote to the editor of *Mother India*, "It is a very good treatment. You can follow it with my blessings."

Cataract and Eye Education

What is cataract? The doctor said, "The eye, just like a camera, has a transparent lens. When somehow the lens shows signs of opacity in its substance then this condition is called cataract."

It was a shock and a matter of great anxiety to me when the doctors at Madras diagnosed early cataract in my eyes and asked me to wait till the cataract was matured for an operation. Though after the operation cataract patients usually become all right yet sometimes the patient suffers much after the operation and in some cases the vision is lost. However, I did not like the idea of an operation and in a depressed state returned to Pondicherry. Next day I consulted Dr. Agarwal in his eye clinic, his reputation for curing eye troubles is prevalent in the Ashram. At first he put some questions regarding my eye trouble and physical fitness. My eyesight had started deteriorating by proof reading in bright electric light and the number of glasses was frequently increased. When I questioned why the number of glasses was increased so often, Dr. Agarwal said that due to strain in reading hypermetropia had developed. My last prescription of glasses was of + 5 for reading. Even with such a high power of glasses my vision was gradually failing, the eyes tired quickly and the vision became hazy, headache and strain increased in reading. Then after a thorough examination in the dark room the doctor said that this kind of a cataract was due to strain hence preventable and curable and there was nothing to worry about. If I could undergo his treatment faithfully for some months, the cataract would dissolve and the vision will improve. I felt very happy and consented to take the treatment. For six months I was regularly attending the eye clinic and doing different eye exercises. I enjoyed the sun treatment and palming and I played with a tennis ball to practise football swing. In this exercise the ball is moved forward with the foot and as it rolled forward the ground appeared to move backward. This observation of apparent movement greatly helped my eyes to relax their muscles. And by doing this exercise in relaxation my physical health also improved. My diet was also regulated.

When I looked at the candle flame while counting 100 respirations I felt as if I had gone into a trance, there was peace in the head and in the nerves of the body. The eyes felt a sort of power in them. I knew Yogis used to concentrate on the candle flame and they maintained good eyesight.

For two months I had completely discarded glasses and allowed my eyes to accommodate themselves in different conditions of life. Then Dr. Agarwal advised me to use glasses of less power and practise with them the methods of eye education in reading. So daily I read small print with glasses in good light as well as in candle light. After six months I found that my eyesight had become normal with glasses and all the discomforts had been chased away. It became quite convenient to read and see proofs for hours. Now two years have passed and I maintain good eyesight and daily devote some time to eye exercises because preservation of good eyesight is impossible without eye education. When Dr. Agarwal re-examined my eyes in the dark room with his instrument, he found no trace of cataract. And such a good condition of eyes I shall maintain now by eye education.

CHANDRADIP

Questions and Answers

A Minister to Government of India consults Dr. Agarwal.

N. I want to consult you, doctor.

D. *Tell me what is your trouble.*

N. Doctors suspect glaucoma and advise me to get my eyes examined every three months for a check-up.

D. *Suppose the trouble is increased, will they be able to prevent it or cure it?*

N. No, they will advise pilocarpine drops.

D. *Why do they suspect glaucoma?*

N. They find cupping in the optic disc; otherwise the eyes are quite normal.

D. *How did your eye trouble start?*

N. Three years back, I was getting attacks of temporary blindness. At times there was a pricking pain also but the doctors found my eyes quite all right.

D. *What is the trouble at present?*

N. At present there is no trouble but about a month back I was getting severe pain and headache; usually in the morning after sleep I felt very uncomfortable. Can you tell me what is the cause of my trouble?

D. *Do you know that your memory is also affected?*

N. Yes, I know.

D. *Don't you feel uncomfortable with your glasses?*

N. Yes, they hurt my eyes but I use them as the doctors have advised me to do so.

D. *Can you read this fine print in this electric light?*

N. I can read but don't feel comfortable.

D. *How do you find reading in candle light?*

N. Fine print is clear and it is soothing and comfortable to read it in candle light.

D. *The cause of your trouble is reading and working for long hours under a bright electric light.*

N. Is it bad to read under a bright light? All along I have been working and reading under a bright light.

D. *Reading under a bright light can do much harm. I shall show you two cases who have suffered a lot by reading for long hours under a high power electric light.*

N. Yes, I have read your articles in *Mother India* where you have recommended reading fine print in dim light or candle light at a close distance, but all these ideas are quite opposite to the general belief.

D. *Those who advise to read big print at an arm's length and in bright light are persons who are above forty. At this age the capacity to read fine print in dim light is lost, so they advise thus, otherwise reading fine print in candle light is extremely beneficial while reading large print under bright light is extremely harmful.*

N. It is said that glaucoma makes the person blind.

D. *Many lose their sight in spite of all medical aid. But all these cases are curable in the early stage by eye education and mental relaxation. And all can be saved from blindness.*

N. When I had trouble, one doctor found the tension just above normal, but after some days another doctor found it below normal.

D. The former doctor examined you when you were having eye trouble, the eyes were under a strain. The other doctor examined your eyes when the trouble was over.

N. That is right. But tell me one thing frankly, "Can you prevent and cure my trouble?

D. Yes, in a week's time you can be all right and the eyes will become immune to future attacks.

N. Thank you very much. I will surely undergo your treatment.

CHAPTER IX
LIMITS OF VISION

It is said that letters on the Snellen Test Card marked twenty
cannot be seen at a greater distance than twenty or thirty feet,
but some persons can read even smaller letters at this distance.
It can be demonstrated that the small letter O with a white
centre can be seen perfectly at any distance when one can
imagine the white centre perfectly white at that distance.
When one can imagine such a letter at thirty feet, his vision will
be 30/10. The perfect imagination of the letter O, or of other
objects, is always associated with perfect sight of other letters
or objects not known.

FIELD. In many cases of imperfect sight not only is central
vision lowered, but there is a loss of the ability to see objects
off to one side. Perfect imagination is a cure for an imperfect
field. In some cases of destruction of the centre of sight of the
retina, with total or partial loss of vision, it is difficult to
understand how the use of perfect imagination or relaxation
has been followed by a permanent cure.

NIGHT BLINDNESS. Some cases with imperfect sight
see better in a bright light than they do in a dim light, and
some cases are so marked that they have been described as
cases of night blindness. These cases are cured at first temporarily, later more continuously by the perfect imagination
of the letter O or some other objects as well as in a dim light
as in a bright light.

DAY BLINDNESS. Some patients may read in good

light only two lines of the Snellen Test Card, but after the light is dimmed, the vision may become 20/10. These cases are quite readily cured by the intelligent use of sun gazing. When the patient becomes able to imagine letters in a bright light as well as in a dim light, the vision becomes normal.

COLOUR BLINDNESS. All persons with imperfect sight have an imperfect perception of colours. They may see large letters blacker than small letters, or the white spaces of large letters may appear whiter than the white spaces of small letters. Some patients may describe the colour of large letters of the Snellen Test Card as blood-red, or they may see the large and small letters as grey or blue or purple, or any colour. The perfect imagination of one letter or other object is a cure for these cases of colour blindness. Even cases of colour blindness associated with diseases of retina or of optic nerve are benefited by the intelligent use of the imagination.

SIZE. The size of letters of the Snellen Test Card or of other objects depends entirely upon the imagination. If the imagination is perfect, one may imagine the size of known or unknown letters at the near point or at the distance correctly. If the imagination is imperfect, the size of letters or other objects will be imagined incorrectly. It is interesting to observe that artists who are familiar with the size of things which they draw, very seldom present a perfect drawing of one object. A portrait painted by one painter may look entirely different from a portrait of the same person by some other artist. It is because of the variation of their imagination.

TREATMENT. It can be demonstrated that we see not the

image focussed upon the retina, but our interpretation or our imagination of this image. Imagination, when used properly, is the most satisfactory, most accurate, most helpful method to obtain perfect sight. To improve the imagination it is first necessary to improve the memory; to improve the memory it is first necessary to improve the sight; to improve the sight it is first necessary to improve the imagination.

HALOS. For example, persons with good sight appear to see the white spaces between the lines of fine print to be whiter than the margin of the page. It can be demonstrated that this is an illusion. We do not see illusions; we only imagine them. When the white spaces between the lines appear whiter than the margin of the page, we call these white spaces halos. Most of us believe we see them, and it is very difficult for many people to realize that the halos are not seen but only imagined. The halos might be called the connecting link between imagination and sight. To see the halos is to improve the imagination, and the vision for the letters is also improved. One can improve the vision for reading not by looking at the letters, but by improvng the imagination of the halos. To look at the letters very soon brings on a strain, with imperfect sight. To look at the white spaces and to improve their whiteness, is a benefit to the imagination and to the vision. One cannot read fine print unless the halos are imagined. By practice one becomes able to imagine or to see the halos more perfectly — the better the imagination, the better the sight.

Concentration and Relaxation

What is concentration? The dictionary says concentration is an effort to keep the mind fixed on a point or to fix the gaze on one point or on one letter or an object. Such a thing is impossible and always causes great strain and those who practise it suffer from imperfect sight and mental strain, and then lose the power of concentration. Their memory, imagination and sight are affected. For example, concentrate your mind and eyes on a part of a big letter of the Snellen Test Card at ten feet, the gaze is fixed at one point. Within a few minutes you will observe that the vision begins to blur, the strain in the eyes and mind becomes evident.

But if by concentration you mean, doing or seeing one thing better than anything else, and shifting the sight from one part to another, then you may speak of concentration: it is then central fixation. For example, look at a small letter on the Snellen Test Card and shift the sight from side to side, observe that the letter appears to make short movements from side to side and the part regarded appears best. This kind of concentration is immensely beneficial to the mind and eyes.

Recent psychology gives a new interpretation to concentration. Attention underlies concentration. The state of attention which seems to be continuous is in reality intermittent; the object of attention is merely a centre, the point to which attention returns again and again. All parts of the objects, and then the reflections inspired by these various parts hold our interest by turns. Even when the attention is fixed on the most trifling material object, it works in just the same fashion. This is entirely according to central fixation as described by Dr. Bates.

There are two aspects of concentration — voluntary and involuntary. Voluntary concentration is an effort and cannot be maintained without fatigue; our thought holds the object in focus. Whereas in involuntary concentration there is no effort, the object holds our thought without our volition as in contemplation and meditation or in central fixation.

Involuntary concentration and relaxation are the same thing. Relaxation of the passive kind usually ends in sleep or sleepiness, as experienced by many patients in palming. Relaxation combined with action as usually one experiences in swinging, central fixation and white line of fine print is also free from effort and strain when done properly.

Another thing about relaxation: obstacles to relaxation may prove sources of relaxation. An instance of which is found in the noise that is keeping us awake when wishing to go to sleep. If we sufficiently relax, if we accept the disturbance and sleep in spite of it, not only is the obstacle overcome, but, because overcome, it in turn becomes rather pleasantly associated with going to sleep. When again we desire to sleep, we find the noise soothing rather than annoying, and really a source of relaxation instead of an obstacle to it.

How to Concentrate

To remember the letter O of fine print continuously and without effort proceed as follows:

Imagine a little black spot on the right-hand side of the O blacker than the rest of the letter; then imagine a similar spot on the left-hand side. Shift the attention from the right-hand spot to the left, and observe that every time you think of the left spot the O appears to move to the right, and every time you think of the right one it appears to move to the left. This motion, when the shifting is done properly, is very short, less than the width of the letter. Later you may become able to imagine the O without conscious shifting and swinging, but whenever the attention is directed to the matter these things will be noticed.

Now do the same thing with a letter on the test card. If the shifting is normal, it will be noted that the letter can be regarded indefinitely, and that it appears to have a slight motion.

To demonstrate that the attempt to concentrate spoils the memory, or imagination, and the vision:

Try to think continuously of a spot on one part of an imagined letter. The spot and the whole letter will soon disappear. Or try to imagine the whole letter, equally black and distinct at one time; this will be found to be even more difficult.

Do the same with a letter on the test card. The results will be the same.

Practical Suggestion

It has been demonstrated that the continuous memory, imagination, or vision of one thing for any length of time is impossible. To see one letter of the Snellen Test Card continuously, it is necessary to shift from one part of the letter to another. By alternately moving the eyes from one side of the letter to the other, it is possible to imagine the letter to be moving in the opposite direction to the movement of the eyes. This movement of the letter is called a swing. When it is slow, easy, short, about one-quarter of an inch or less, maximum vision is obtained which continues as long as the swing continues.

As long as we are awake, we are thinking, remembering, or imagining mental pictures, and are comfortable. To go around blind requires a distinct effort which is a strain on all the nerves and is always uncomfortable. The normal mind alternates its attention from one mental picture to another, which is a relaxation or rest. The memory, or imagination, is best when one thing is imagined better than all other things, and this is Central Fixation, but constant shifting is necessary to maintain Central Fixation.

One of the best methods to improve the vision is to regard a letter of the Snellen Test Card with the eyes open, then close the eyes and remember or imagine the letter better for about ten seconds, then open the eyes for a moment. By alternately regarding the letter with the eyes open and closed, the imagination of the letter improves in flashes. By continuing to alternate the flashes improve and last longer until the vision becomes continuously improved.

Brain Tension

The brain has many nerves. Part of these nerves are called ganglion cells and originate in some particular part of the brain. Each has a function of its own. They are connected with other ganglion cells and with the aid of nerve fibres are connected with others located in various parts of the brain as well as in the spinal cord, the eye, the ear, the nerve of smell, taste, and the nerves of touch. The function of each ganglion cell of the brain is different from that of all others. When the ganglion cells are healthy, they function in a normal manner.

The retina of the eye contains numerous ganglion cells which regulate special things such as normal vision, normal memory, normal imagination and they do this with a control more or less accurate of other ganglion cells of the whole body. The retina has a similar structure to parts of the brain. It is connected to the brain by the optic nerve.

Many nerves from the ganglion cells of the retina carry conscious and unconscious control of other ganglion cells which are connected to other parts of the body.

When the ganglion cells are diseased or at fault, the function of all parts of the body are not normally maintained. In all cases of imperfect sight, it has been repeatedly demonstrated that the ganglion cells and nerves of the brain are under a strain. When this strain is corrected by treatment, the function of the ganglion and other cells becomes normal. The importance of mental treatment cannot be over-estimated.

A study of the facts has demonstrated that a disease of some ganglion in any part of the body occurs in a similar ganglion in the brain.

Brain tension of one or more nerves always means disease of the nerve ganglia. Treatment of the mind with the aid of sight, memory and imagination has cured many cases of imperfect sight without other treatment.

Diseases of the Retina

It is a common belief that optic neuritis or optic atrophy is mostly due to syphilitic or some other infection in the system or bad teeth. The following facts are to be considered:

1. Many people suffer from syphilis or some other infection but very very few suffer from optic neuritis, and those who suffer from optic neuritis are usually not benefited by anti-syphilitic treatment or anti-toxin treatment or by extraction of teeth.

2. Some cases of optic neuritis do not give any indication, by tests or otherwise, of syphilis or toxin or bad teeth.

3. Some cases of optic neuritis whether they suffer from any infection or not recover partially or completely by themselves by rest without any specific treatment.

How can these facts be reconciled with each other if syphilis or some other infection is the cause of optic neuritis?

A patient had developed optic neuritis in the left eye and all the possible tests were made to find out the source of infection but the result was negative. He could hardly see the top letter of the chart from one foot and could not perceive colours. The expression of the face indicated that the eye was under a great strain. By eye education and relaxation he was completely cured.

Facts Reconciled

The primary cause of optic neuritis is eye strain and mental strain. If the strain already exists syphilis or any other infection may exaggerate the strain and consequently may cause more damage, but they themselves can hardly cause optic neuritis or optic atrophy when there is proper relaxation of the mind and eyes. That is why patients suffering from syphilis or other infection may remain free from optic neuritis, and anti-syphilitic or anti-toxin treatment in positive cases may do no good. Cases who recover themselves without any specific treatment or by some specific treatment indicate that somehow the strain was relieved from the eyes and mind. Treatment of strain, side by side, with other treatments of any infection will prove really beneficial; but drastic treatment should be avoided as far as possible.

Q: If the trouble is due to strain, then how is it that one eye may be affected and the other remains free, as in the above case?

A: This is because one has two separate eyes — one may function under a strain and the other not.

Q: Why do not all persons suffering from mental strain suffer from optic neuritis or some such eye trouble?

A: If the mind is under a strain, but if the eyes do not make an effort to see, the person will remain free from all such eye troubles; but if the mind is under a strain and the eye also stares, imperfect sight will be the result. The habitual strain may cause diseases of the eye — functional as well as organic.

Q: *Then why does anti-syphilitic or anti-toxin treatment help considerably in certain cases, if the strain is the main cause?*

A: Syphilis or any other infection might be increasing the strain of the mind and eyes, hence anti-syphilitic treatment or anti-toxin treatment helped such cases. Or these cases might be recovering in a natural course of relaxation and anti-toxin treatment got the credit.

Floating Specks

When a patient stares or strains to see by looking at a light-coloured surface he may see, or imagine he sees, floating black specks, strings of black thread or small light-coloured globules resembling tears. The floating specks may be apparently a quarter of an inch or more in size and they may be of any shape.

Many nervous people have been made very unhappy by seeing these floating specks. The cause of floating specks is strain or an imperfect memory of perfect sight. Persons with normal vision can be taught how to imagine them by straining.

In the treatment of floating specks it is important to convince the patients that they are unreal, they are only imagined and not seen. It helps much to impress on the patient's mind that to see these floating specks requires a sufficient strain.

Frequent palming, long swing and central fixation exercises

are very helpful to cure the trouble of floating specks. Two more instructions are necessary:

1. Whenever floating specks appear, ignore and shift sight to near.

2. Never experiment whether they are visible or not.

A doctor friend can see consciously at will, any time he desires, floating specks. He notices the strain in the eyes at that time. On taking the sight away from the floating specks and paying no attention to them and giving the eyes some rest, they are no longer seen.

(Details of floating specks from *Secrets of Indian Medicine*)

Threatened Blindness and Floating Specks

"Most of the patients who attend the School for Perfect Eyesight at Pondicherry to consult Dr. Agarwal are usually chronic and so-called incurable. When they do not get any relief in their eye troubles from other doctors, then they try relaxation treatment which is so successfully going on in the clinical department of this School.

"I had the habit to read under powerful electric light up to the middle of the night. Gradually some difficulties regarding my eyesight began to develop and created difficulty to see properly when I came from light to darkness and *vice versa*. Later on I began to see floating specks before my eyes and this became very annoying. My distant vision also became weak. Then my father took me to the Cuttuck Medical College for a thorough check-up. There many doctors examined my eyes and it was discovered that my retina had degenerated and it was declared that there were chances of becoming blind in future. Such a prognosis was a shock to me and to my parents. Many injections and tablets were tried to improve the blood circulation and vitality but all that was in vain. At this time my uncle Shree Manoj Das of Sri Aurobindo Ashram wrote to my father that he had not seen until now any case who had not improved under the care of Dr. Agarwal. My father intuitively felt he should take me to Pondicherry for treatment.

"Doctors at Cuttuck had failed to find any cause for my eye trouble in spite of various tests. When my father asked Dr. Agarwal about the cause the doctor said that it was due to great strain on the eyes while reading for long hours under high power electric light. Constant reflection from the paper had affected the retina. Other factors such as constipation, poor action of the liver had helped the trouble to increase.

"Dr. Agarwal gave good hope of improvement after thorough examination of my eyes. The first thing that he taught me to relieve the strain was blinking. I had developed the habit of staring while reading or seeing things at a distance. During treatment I was reminded by the doctor whenever I did not blink or did winking instead of blinking. By correct blinking floating specks have almost disappeared but when I unconsciously begin to stare, they appear and remind me to blink. Frequently I do palming for ten or fifteen minutes at a time and this relaxes my eyes and mind and the nerves of the whole body. Reading fine print in good light and in candle light alternately has greatly helped me to read ordinary print without any strain. At the end of different exercises such as swinging and central fixation my eyes are bandaged for half an hour with some medicine upon them. On every Monday I take an enema. My diet has been regulated with more fruits and greens.

"Regarding floating specks Dr. Agarwal gave two important instructions. One is to ignore them when they appear. The other is: do not experiment to see them when they are not present.

"The result of all this treatment seems to me very wonderful. My health and vision have considerably improved. I have discarded my goggles and spectacles and am no more afraid of threatening blindness, I enjoy good eyesight, my mind and eyes are quite relaxed. It is hoped that one day Orissa also will have such an eye clinic for the cure of imperfect eyes without glasses."

SIDDHARTHA DAS

Retinitis Pigmentosa

Almost every eye specialist is of opinion that there is no treatment for Retinitis Pigmentosa and that the patient would become blind in due course of time. What is retinitis pigmentosa?

In retinitis pigmentosa some black spots form on the surface of the retina. Patient usually complains of gradual loss of vision, night blindness and contraction of field of vision. The disease usually occurs in females.

Recently three lady patients, married, having children quite normal, attended the School for Perfect Eyesight. On examination it was clearly revealed that they were suffering from Retinitis Pigmentosa. Their mind was under a great fear that they would become blind sooner or later as suggested by many eye specialists. Due to the fear of becoming blind they were in search of some one who could save them from blindness.

We observed some very important phenomena in these cases. In one case the retina was full of many pigments but the vision was almost normal both for distance and near. In another case the pigments were much less yet the vision was greatly affected. In the third case, a doctor's wife, there were only a few pigments but the night blindness and contraction of field of vision were prominent. Now the question is why was there no loss of vision and no night blindness when the pigments were many in the first case?

Vision is a process of mental interpretation of retinal images. Our vision mostly depends on the power of the mental interpretation. We found that this case had a normal expression of the face; otherwise usually cases of retinitis pigmentosa express a peculiar facial expression indicating great strain on the mind and eyes. Her memory and imagination were very good. In palming she could easily observe perfect darkness before the eyes.

Almost all cases of retinitis pigmentosa show good improvement by sun treatment, palming and central fixation. All these three lady patients improved their eyesight and general health of their eyes. The fear of becoming blind had fled away from their consciousness. Their gratitude was immense.

Questions and Answers

Q: I told a doctor friend about your good treatment for defective vision and blindness but he simply ridiculed the whole thing. Why?

A: Many doctors have still not developed the true scientific attitude. They follow conventional authority like a religionist who sticks to some particular dogmas. A true scientist is always willing to make new experiments and accept new truths.

Q: What was the trouble with Rajesh whose right eye was almost blind due to an injury from a tennis-ball?

A: The eye in appearance was all right but had lost its proper functioning, so by relaxation of the eye and mind through some exercises the eye began to function and now he can read the smallest type.

Q: *What is the cause of defective eyesight?*

A: All defective vision is due to strain in some form, and strain is relieved by relaxation.

You can demonstrate to your satisfaction that strain lowers the vision. When you stare, you strain. Look fixedly at one object for five seconds or longer. What happens? The object blurs and finally disappears. Also, your eyes are made uncomfortable by this experiment. When you rest your eyes for a few moments the vision is improved and the discomfort relieved.

Q: *I am forty-five. My eyesight for distance is quite good but my reading sight is failing. What should I do?*

A: Concentrate on a candle flame for a few minutes, then do palming and read some small type at any convenient distance and gradually bring the print nearer to the eyes.

CHAPTER X

SEVEN TRUTHS OF NORMAL SIGHT

1. Normal sight can always be demonstrated in the normal eye, but only under favourable conditions.

2. CENTRAL FIXATION: The letter or part of the letter regarded is always seen best.

3. SHIFTING: The point regarded changes rapidly and continuously.

4. SWINGING: When the shifting is slow, the letters appear to move from side to side, or in other directions with a pendulum-like motion.

5. MEMORY IS PERFECT: The colour and background of the letters or other objects seen, are remembered perfectly, instantaneously and continuously.

6. IMAGINATION IS GOOD: One may even see the white part of letters whiter than it really is, while the black is not altered by distance, illumination, size, or form of the letters.

7. REST OR RELAXATION OF THE EYE AND MIND is perfect and can always be demonstrated.
   When one of these seven fundamentals is perfect, all are perfect.
   (For details consult *Mind & Vision*)

When the sight is imperfect, these facts are not observed or are observed partly. If somehow they can be produced in the defective eye, the sight would become normal and this suggests the cure. If one is able to observe them perfectly at 3 ft. the sight is normal at 3 ft., and if one is able to note at 20 ft., the sight is normal at 20 ft., and so on.

Blinking Education

1. Observe what is blinking and what is winking. Then do palming and recall the memory of blinking. Then take a mirror, shift sight from one eye to the other, blink at each shift.

2. Hold your index fingers, one at six inches from the face, other at arm's length. Shift the sight from one finger to the other. This will give you the idea how much movement the lids should make in blinking.

3. Take a ball, move it from side to side, 100 movements, blink at each side.

4. Take a ball, throw it up, about 1 ft. to 2 ft. high, move the head and not the lids, with the movement of the ball.

5. Walk, blink at each step.

6. Shift the sight on white lines and blink at each line.

7. Count irregularly and blink at each count.

8. Put two candles one foot apart, blink at each flame with the movement of respirations.

9. When typing, blink often.

10. Blink, when you inhale and exhale.

Proper Use of the Eyes

READING—Shift the sight and blink gently and hold the book at 10 or 12 inches.

2. WRITING — Shift the sight with the movement of the pen and blink. To develop this habit:
   a. Draw straight lines horizontally or vertically.
   b. Draw angular lines and circular lines.
   c. Write letters or dictation.
   d. Cover what you write.

3. CINEMA — Keep the eyes half open and blink. Staring or intent look is harmful. Avoid seeing advertisements. Palm during the interval.

4. SEWING — Shift the sight with the movement of the needle.

5. TRAVELLING — Train — Observe trees and poles moving backwards while far distant objects appear to move forward. Keeping the sight fixed on one object causes strain.

6. DRIVING — Observe the side objects moving backwards or the road gliding backwards or shift the sight from the road to the speedometer or flag of the car.

7. CYCLING — Observe the road and side objects moving backwards.

8. BUS — Look at the movements of the conductor or the objects moving backwards. Avoid reading the signboards or fixing the sight on some objects.

9. BOATING — observe water moving backwards and distant land objects moving forward or look at the movements of the boatman.

10. SHOPPING — Avoid seeing each and every shop and

signboard. Go to the required shop while blinking.

11. LIFT — Look at the operator and side things will appear gliding backwards.

Sun Treatment

1. SUN TREATMENT WITH EYES CLOSED

a. In a chair, make a movement from side to side.

b. In a rocking chair, make a movement forward and backward.

c. Imagine a shifting from one knee to the other.

d. Take a ball, make a movement from side to side in the hands.

2. USE OF SUNGLASS OR MAGNIFYING LENS

a. On closed eyelids, a movement from side to side.

b. Condensing rays on the white part, the sclera, when the patient looks downwards, make a quick movement.

3. OPEN EYE SUN TREATMENT

a. Shift sight below the sun when not hot.

b. Stand in the sea or a river or keep feet in cold water and glance at the sun with frequent blinking.

4. SUN TREATMENT FOR BABIES

Sway the baby gently from side to side.

5. SUN TREATMENT BELOW A TREE

When the sun is too hot or unbearable.

6. WHEN THE SUN NOT AVAILABLE

Take the help of a 200 or 500 watt lamp.

7. SUN TREATMENT ALONG WITH EYE-WASH

Fill the basin with cold water to which salt may be added; dip the eyes and face in the water and then glance at the sun with blinking; repeat about ten times.

Short Notes on Palming

1. a. Hands crossed, elbows on a cushion
   b. Palms sideways, elbows resting on a table
   c. Palming with wet palms or wet cotton in palms
   d. One hand palming while rolling a ball with the other.
2. a. Imagine something interesting.
   b. Imagination of a black object, coal-tar, ink, velvet.
   c. Imagine as if stitching a white ribbon on black velvet.
3. a. Imagination of a game or any familiar object or
   b. Palming while counting 100 respirations or
   c. Palming while hearing music or singing a song or
   d. Imagination of sense of smell or touch.
4. WRONG PALMING
   a. Legs crosswise and uncomfortable posture.
   b. Pressure on the eye-balls and light entering the eyes.
   c. Effort to imagine black.
5. EFFECTS OF SUCCESSFUL PALMING
   a. Improvement in eyesight and feeling of relaxation.
   b. Relief of pain or any other discomfort or strain.
   c. Sense of coolness in the head.
6. EXPERIENCE WHILE PALMING
   a. Perfect darkness before the eyes.
   b. Printer's ink is the standard of black.
   c. Less black or any other colour is the sign of unsuccessful palming.
7. HOW TO HELP IN UNSUCCESSFUL CASES

a. Develop memory equal to sight by glancing at a letter
for a second then closing the eyes for a few seconds till
the memory is equal to sight.
b. Practise central fixation, then palming.
c. Face a blank surface, recall your signature.

Candle Practices

1. CONCENTRATION
   a. Concentrate on the flame while counting 100 respirations.
   b. While concentrating keep the imagination of the flame
in the heart or mind.
   c. With both eyes and each eye — count 25 respirations.
   d. Shift sight from side to side of the flame; then the
flame appears to move in the opposite direction.

2. WHITE LINE
   a. Shift sight on the white lines of Photo Print or Fine Print
with blinking in candle-light.
   b. Shift sight on white lines in good light and candle-light
alternative — 3 times.

3. READING IN CANDLE-LIGHT
   a. Reading of Fundamentals or Fine Print or
   b. Reading of Photo print.
   c. Reading in good light and candle-light alternately.
   d. Read and glance at the blank surface alternately.

4. CENTRAL FIXATION IN CANDLE-LIGHT
   a. On Om Chart — Shift sight on the angular lines.
   b. Snellen Chart — top and bottom or side to side.
   c. On Fundamentals or any reading matter — each word
appearing darker.

5. SWINGING

Put 2 candles nine inches apart, shift sight from one candle to the other and observe that the candles appear to move in the opposite direction.

Alternate Eye Exercises After Palming

1. Central fixation on the eye chart in hand or at 3 feet in good light, and reading 3 pages in dim light keeping the book at a distance from where it is difficult to read, that is, with strain. Alternate. This is useful in myopia.

2. Read Fundamentals in good light and eye chart at 15 or 20 ft. The chart should be in dim light so that the eye may feel strain to see the letters. Alternate. Useful in Hypermetropia or Presbyopia.

3. Long swing 100 and white line in Fine Print or Photo Print with gentle blinking. Alternate. Useful in astigmatism.

4. Run around a chair, 5 rounds, and read the chart at 5 ft. to 10 ft. This running around a chair may be done with a ball so that interest is created. Instead of the chart Fundamentals may be given. Useful for children.

5. Long swing and concentration on flame, alternately: Concentration on flame may be with 25 or 50 or 100 respirations. The sight is on the flame but concentration is on respirations. Useful in hypermetropia or presbyopia especially.

6. Alternate reading of Fine Print and palming, 3 times.

7. Long swing and central fixation on chart. Alternate.

8. Sewing 20 stitches and reading the chart at 10 ft. Alternate.

9.   Reading Fundamentals or Fine Print in good light and candle light. Alternate.

10.   Walking with blinking at each step and reading Fine Print or the chart at 10 ft. Alternate.

11.   Football swing. Sight moves with the ball, the ground appears to move backwards. Read Photo Print.

12.   Variable swing and reading Fine Print in candle light. Alternate.

Games of Eyesight

1. FAST PRACTICE: Different eye education exercises are arranged, participants move from one exercise to another as the bell rings every two minutes or every five minutes.

Exercises for selection — Long swing, variable swing, shoulder swing, palming, sewing, writing, painting, filling white centres of letters of a newspaper, filling dots in a half-inch circle, concentration on candle flame while counting 100 respirations, reading in candle-light, white lines in Fine Print, Central Fixation on Om Chart.

2. MERRY-GO-ROUND AND CANDLE FLAME: Five participants move around a stool on which a candle is put, they sing and then sit and read Fine Print or Photo Print. Repeat.

3. GAME OF COMMONEY: This game is very helpful to teach new terminology. Name is given to each participant, for example, Retina, myopia, hypermetropia, astigmatism, presbyopia, lens, iris, cornea, macula, pupil, eye-balls etc. The captain tells a story referring to those names. Hearing the particular name the participant stands up, makes a round and sits down. When COMMONEY is called, then all stand and make a round and sit down.

4. MUSICAL CHAIRS: One chair less than the number of participants. Different eye exercises are arranged by the side of the chairs. For example:

Central Fixation on chart, reading Fundamentals, reading Fine Print, blinking on white lines, reading in candle-light, blinking in a mirror, blinking with the help of two index fingers, circular swing with the help of the finger movement, reading the chart at a distance, writing letters of the chart, writing Fundamentals or Fine Print matter, memory swing, etc.

Participants move around the chairs while bouncing the balls; when the bell rings, they sit down and practise the exercise.

Treatment Chart

School For Perfect Eyesight

Ref. No. 867   *Dated* 2-9-70
....
Name Krishna
....

Take the following treatment morning and evening:

1. First apply the medicine   Resolvent 200
    with a rod in each eye.

2. After the application of the medicine, sit facing the sun
    with the eyes closed for about 5 minutes. While taking
    the sun treatment, move the body gently from side to side
    like a pendulum.

3. After sun treatment come to the shade and wash the eyes
    with water and Ophthalmo.

4. Now sit comfortably with the eyes closed and covered

with palms (palming) for about 5 minutes.

After palming, practise the following with both eyes and with each eye separately.

Long swing 50 to 100 or Central Fixation on chart in hand.

Concentration on candle flame while counting 100 respirations.

Read Fundamentals or Fine Print in good light and candle-light.

Get the habit of blinking, avoid staring. Adopt any other exercise which suits you most.

Take a record of vision before starting the treatment.

Read the Snellen Eye Chart before going to school.

School for Perfect Eyesight

In the course of his development, man has discovered various means for the prevention and cure of diseases. The chief among them are Ayurveda, Allopathy and Homeopathy. In recent times, Dr. Bates developed the knowledge of the cure of defective eyesight. He noted that the eye and mind were under a strain in all the various types of defective eyesight and eye troubles. He, therefore, developed methods of eye education and mental relaxation. Dr. Bates has made many remarkable discoveries regarding accommodation of the eye and errors of refraction. Even with regard to so-called incurable cases, his methods of treatment bring quick improvement in eyesight and relieve pain and discomfort.

One of the aims of the Sri Aurobindo International Centre of Education is to promote a new synthesis of knowledge, and in this attempt a synthesis of various systems of medicine plays an important part. The School for Perfect Eye Sight is one of the experiments in this direction, with Dr. Bates as the main scientific path-pointer. It was opened on May 5, 1968 with the profound message of the Divine Mother:

"THE MORE THE MIND IS QUIET THE MORE THE SIGHT IS GOOD."

The School provides a course in Ophthalmic Science which will not be limited to any particular system of medicine but will draw from all systems and even attempt a fresh inquiry on new lines. The duration of this course will normally be of four years and the pre-requisite for admission to this course will be a good knowledge of English and an interest in pursuing the course.

All along it has been my experience that mental relaxation is the key of success in life, in Yoga and in education. Under the present civilised conditions man's mind is under a severe strain, hence preservation of good eyesight is almost impossible without eye education and mental relaxation. In this direction *Mother India* has done a great service to educate the mind of the public. Many enquiries have come and many have attended the School. Often it is a surprise how quickly the vision begins to improve by simple methods of eye education. One girl student, Dolia, from our Centre of Education, whose eyesight had failed both for far and near, recovered normal eyesight in about a week's time. Our Registrar Mr. Kireet Joshi was surprised when he found that reading Fine Print in dim light or candle light improved his eyesight and produced good relaxation.

It is hoped that our future doctors will integrate all the systems of medicine harmoniously and bring quick recovery by their simple and harmless methods. At a later stage this School for Perfect Eyesight may be shifted to Auroville where it will be joined to the World University and will become a unique institution in the world, imparting medical knowledge to bring perfection not only in eyesight but in the body as a whole and in the mind's general functions.

Exhibition of Eye Education at the School

It was towards the end of the nineteenth century that in America Dr. W. H. Bates was born. He was a distinguished pioneer in Ophthalmology and developed a new system of eye education.

Some of the pictures show how the eye should be used while reading, writing, sewing, spinning, in the cinema and during various activities of life. In other illustrations in this group Dr. Bates recommends three most important things:

1. Reading Fine Print is a benefit to the eye while large print is a menace.

2. Reading in dim light or in candle light is very useful.

3. Reading at a closer distance is beneficial.

Dr. Bates admits that India has many secrets: for example, Sun Treatment as shown in a picture. Facing the sun with eyes closed for a few minutes gives health and vitality to the eyes. Palming is a sort of meditation which brings wonderful relaxation to the mind and to the nerves and helps to improve the eyesight. Children respond very well and usually give surprising results.

In one picture Dr. R. S. Agarwal is giving a demonstration on eye education. Recently a teacher of the Centre of Education, whose left eye was blind from childhood, got cured. A doll represents the blind eye case and tells people to join the one year training course in eye education. Now we enter into the classroom where the furniture has been fitted in the form of the Mother's symbol — in the centre a flower-stand, four tables around it complete the circle, twelve chairs are around the tables. On the book-rack about 12 publications by Dr. Agarwal in English and in Indian languages indicate that much work has been done in India on the lines of Dr. Bates.

In the first picture here the structural condition of the eye-ball is shown when the eye is Hypermetropic, Normal and Myopic. In the second diagram is shown the construction of the eye and how the eye looks from inside when examined by an instrument called the Ophthalmoscope. The illustrations on Accommodation are very interesting. One of them proves that focusing at a near point is brought about by the action of the oblique muscles of the eye and not by increased curvature of the lens. The other picture shows that the eye and the camera are alike in structure and functioning. The last painting illustrates the vision of the inner eye.

Now we come to the practical side. The two dolls show what blinking is, how gently their lids move in blinking which should not be mistaken for winking. In the dark room one is taught how to read in dim light and in candle light. The sun-lamp is meant for sun treatment when there is no sun. The palming pillows help in Palming. In the medicine room patients learn how to apply Resolvent 200 to improve eye-sight.

Art of Writing

"Doctor, my eyes get tired soon in writing and it becomes difficult to finish even a page. I have not written a letter to my father for a long time due to the pain and headache which manifest when I start writing. Look, I have so many pairs of glasses though I see well, and here are so many medicines prescribed by eminent eye specialists, but none helps to relieve my troubles. This chronic redness persists in my eyes for a long time." This is the story of the princess, the daughter of the Late Maharaja of Nepal, whom I had treated earlier for high myopia.

I found her vision normal both for distance and near. After a little thought, I asked the princess to write something in my presence. After a few lines she stopped as the pain and heaviness had started. I understood the cause of her trouble, so I told her that she would be all right on the third day. She was very happy to hear such words of assurance but questioned the cause of her trouble. I told her that she herself would know during the course of her treatment.

The fact is this, that she had adopted the wrong way of writing. While writing she had the habit of reading the words already written. To correct this wrong habit I advised her to draw straight lines and shift the sight with the movement of the pen. As there was nothing to read she could easily draw lines while shifting the sight with the movement of the pen. Then she began to draw angular lines and then began to write. While writing she used a piece of blotting paper to hide the written matter. Then on the third day she wrote about ten pages without any discomfort and without the help of the blotting paper. To convince her that her trouble was due to improper use of the eyes in writing, I told her to write a page in the wrong way, that is, while writing trying to read the already written words. Very soon she began to feel the discomfort and her handwriting became unsteady. Again she started writing in the right way and she could write pages with ease and comfort, she just shifted the sight with the movement of the pen without any attempt to read the already written words.

See the Natural Way

Khorshed while on educational tour to U.S.A. was experiencing some difficulty in reading and writing. Her eyes quickly tired and became prominent as if protruding from the bony socket, a horrible appearance quite disfiguring to the face. At times while reading the words appeared double and often she made mistakes in transcription. She had to give up the work of stitching as sewing was very uncomfortable. There was a constant feeling of dryness and heaviness in the eyes. Often her lady friends laughed at her inability to match the colours while selecting some cloth. She had developed the habit of staring while reading or seeing different objects. At times the pain and headache became severe and she had to rest long hours. The glare of the sun was very unpleasant and when she moved in an unknown place she got knocks as her field of vision was contracted.

When Khorshed put these visual difficulties before the eye specialists at U.S.A. they found her eyes quite normal. They could not think that these visual defects could be due to mental strain and wrong use of the eyes. They put her to different tests and the conclusion was that her eye troubles were due to Hyperthyrodism. When she returned to India, Bombay doctors supported the diagnosis and treatment of U.S.A. doctors and gave thyroid orally but there was no relief to her eye troubles.

Finally Khorshed left herself at the mercy of the Divine Grace. One morning she was on a visit to Sri Aurobindo Ashram and had an opportunity to visit the School for Perfect Eyesight. She is an intelligent and charming personality hence it was necessary to tell her frankly that it was a mistake of our specialists to collaborate the visual defects with the thyroid disorder. Both were quite separate troubles. Hence the treatment of thyroid failed to give any relief. I explained to her that the eye being a sense organ was closely associated with the mind in its functioning. The strain of the mind would immediately affect the eyesight, while the relaxation of the mind would benefit the eyes. To demonstrate this fact she was asked to stand before a window with vertical bars in it. When she moved the body, head and eyes to the right while raising the left heel she observed that the bars of the window appeared to be moving to the left and vice versa. As soon as she practised this swing in the right way she felt greatly relaxed but when she practised the swing in the wrong way, she felt a great strain in the eyes and head.

Another great difficulty was that she did not blink. She did not know how necessary it was to blink gently to keep the eyes at rest all the time. It was difficult at first to adopt the right habit of blinking but by the application of different relaxation exercises and bandaging she could train her eye lids to blink in a normal way.

When the sight is perfect the subject is able to observe that all objects regarded appear to be moving. A letter seen at the near or at the distance appears to move slightly in various directions. The pavement comes towards the person in walking, and the side houses appear to move in the opposite direction. In reading, the page appears to move in a direction opposite to the movement of the eyes. If one tries to imagine things stationary, the vision is lowered and the discomforts and pain may be produced. By observing the movement of lines while shifting the sight on white lines in between the lines of print, Khorshed felt a great relief and could read and write for a long period without any discomfort. In sewing she shifted the sight with the movement of the needle. To overcome the glare of the sun she faced the sun for a few minutes daily.

Whenever Khorshed looked intently at a letter or an object she felt fatigue and discomfort and the object blurred or became double. There was a feeling of tension in the eyes and head. To break this habit of staring she was taught the following:

1. Shift consciously from one part to another of all objects regarded, and imagine that these objects appeared to move in a direction contrary to the movement of the eye.

2. Look at the blackness of the letter for a second and close the eyes for half a minute while recalling the memory of black. When she practised successfully, the memory of blackness increased. Then she did palming for sufficient time till she felt her eyes greatly relaxed.

3. Looking towards the candle flame while counting one hundred respirations soothed her nerves greatly. While reading Fine Print she moved her body forward and backward.

Go to the Movies

In today's world it is ridiculous to tell the students and others not to go to the movies so that the eyes may not be spoiled. It is a common belief that cinematograph pictures are injurious to the eyes, and it is a fact that at times they cause much discomfort and lowering of the vision. They can, however, be made a means of improving eyesight. When they hurt the eyes it is because the subject strains to see the cinema. If this tendency to strain can be overcome, the vision is always benefited and the discomforts are relieved.

I advise most of the eye-patients to go to the movies frequently, become accustomed to the flickering light and the fluctuations of light and learn to look at the picture without strain. They are advised to keep the upper lids down in the position of rest and to blink frequently. They are warned not to stare. If the picture hurts the eyes I instruct them to look away to the dark for a while, then look at a corner of the picture; and so on. In this way the patients soon become able to look directly at the picture without any discomfort. When this does not help, I ask them to try palming for five minutes or longer, that is, to close the eyes and cover them with the palms avoiding any pressure on the eye-balls and then recall the memory of black colour or the episode.

The fact is that vision under difficult conditions is a good mental training. The mind may be disturbed at first by the unfavourable environment; but after it has become accustomed to such environments, the mental control and, consequently, the eyesight is improved.

I remember a very interesting case whose eyes were greatly hurt whenever she went to see cinema. Each time she saw a movie her eyes had swelling and she had severe headache which was relieved after four hours rest. Under the instructions of a doctor she had stopped seeing movies but this itself was a strain on her mind as she was very fond of seeing the movies. After a few days treatment I asked this lady patient to go to the movies and see the cinema with frequent blinking. Formerly she used to stare at the cinematograph pictures and did not blink at all, so she suffered. At first she was hesitant but when I encouraged her that this will prove very helpful, she went and enjoyed the picture with gentle blinking. At the interval time she palmed her eyes and remembered the episode. I had told her not to see the advertisements. After seeing the picture when she came out of the hall she was telling to her friends how beneficial it was to see the cinema in the right way. There was absolutely no headache and no pain and no swelling in the eyes.

If the children and others are taught about the proper use of the eyes, most of the eye troubles will fade away in a natural way. Preservation of good eyesight is impossible without eye education.

Questions and Answers

Q: When I read big print I feel a strain and discomfort but when I read small print I feel relaxed and comfortable. Why is it so?

A: In reading big print one has to see a larger area at a time and this affects the sensitiveness of the eyes and gives the feeling of strain; while in reading small print one sees a smaller area and this helps the eyes' sensitiveness and so one feels relaxed. When small print can be read in the right way, without any discomfort, it becomes extremely beneficial to the eyes.

Q: You say successful Palming is very effective in relieving strain and headache and in improving eyesight, but when I do Palming I do not see perfect darkness before my eyes. What do you suggest?

A: Look at something black or the Chart letter, then close the eyes and recall the black colour seen. Repeat this several times till the memory and the sight are equal. Then do palming. Continue palming for 15 or 20 minutes.

Q: My eyesight is all right but I cannot read comfortably, the right eye suffers. What to do?

A: Read Fine Print in good light and in candle-light alternately three times, with both eyes and each eye separately.

Q: When I get up in the morning, my eyes open with difficulty,

*at times there is some headache also. And I find my memory
becoming dull.*

A: Before sleep and after sleep practice palming for about
20 minutes.

*Q: How is it that on some days I can see the whole chart but
on other days only a few lines?*

A: When there is no strain the vision is normal. Continuous
practice will make the sight all right on other days too.

*Q: Why is my vision worse on a rainy or cloudy day than in
broad daylight?*

A: Because you strain to see on a dark day. Practise palming more on such days.

*Q: The vision in my son's eyes is failing due to Retinitis Pig-
mentosa. Doctors of India and abroad give no hope and the boy
is supposed to become blind in due course of time. Is there any
hope by your methods?*

A: Yes, your son can improve but cannot be cured.

Q: My eyesight is normal. What should I do to keep it so?

A: Read an Eye-chart at a twenty-feet distance and read
fine print daily.

*Q: If the letters of the Eye-chart can be seen more distinctly
with the eyes partly closed or a little screwed, is it advisable to
read that way?*

A: No, it is not advisable. Look at the letters of the Eye-
chart with gentle blinking.

*Q: Can a patient, while practising your method, carry on his
work as usual?*

A: Yes, most patients continue their work just the same and find time to practise palming several times a day and, during all their activities, they do gentle blinking.

Q: Is looking at the green grass or the blue sky helpful to the eyes?

A: Yes, because there is nothing to stare at.

Q: Instead of palming, can I sit in a dark room or cover my eyes with a black cloth or bandage them?

A: No, it does not serve the purpose of palming.

Q: I am suffering from glaucoma and early cataract. Can your methods help me?

A: If your eyesight is defective apart from these diseases, it can certainly be improved in spite of them. As for these diseases, each case is individual and we have to try out our methods to see what results they may have. According to Dr. Bates, cataract-opacity of a certain kind — one due to contraction of the lens — is curable by his methods of eye-relaxation.

Q: Can you tell me the dates of birth and death of Dr. Bates?

A: Dr. Bates was born on December 23, 1860 and died on July 10, 1931. It is in 1931 that I started the work on Dr. Bates lines.

CHAPTER XI

EYE HYGIENE

According to the accepted ideas of eye hygiene, it is important to protect the eyes from a great variety of influences which are often very difficult to avoid, and when people are under their influence, they are thought to be ruining their eyes. Bright lights, artificial lights, dim lights, sudden fluctuations of light, fine print, reading in moving vehicles, reading lying down, etc., have long been considered "bad for the eyes". These ideas are diametrically opposed to the truth. When the eyes are properly used, vision under adverse conditions becomes an actual benefit, because a greater degree of relaxation is required to see under such conditions than under more favourable ones. It is true that the conditions in question may at first cause discomfort, even to persons with normal vision; but a careful study of the facts has demonstrated that only persons with imperfect sight can seriously suffer from them, and if such persons practise central fixation, they quickly become accustomed to them and derive great benefit from them. Hence persons of defective eyesight ought to be educated to use the eyes properly with gentle blinking under adverse conditions for a greater benefit.

1. Expose the eyes to the morning sun for a few minutes daily to make the eyes strong.

2. Go to the movies to accustom yourself to sudden fluctuations of light. This will prove very useful.

3. Reading in a bright light and dim light alternately, or going from a dark room to a well lighted room, and *vice versa* are very beneficial.

4. Reading Fine Print daily is extremely beneficial.

5. Reading in moving vehicles helps in improving the sight.

6. Reading in a lying posture is very delightful. Anyone who can read lying down without discomfort is not likely to have any difficulty in reading under ordinary conditions.

The fact is that vision under difficult conditions is a good mental training. The mind may be disturbed at first by the unfavourable environment; but after it has become accustomed to such environments, the mental control and the eyesight are improved.

Why Eyes Fail to See

It is a fact that glasses have greatly helped many persons who cannot see well at a distance or near, but this is also true that glasses have become an added torture to increase pain and suffering and loss of sight in many cases. The fast deterioration in eyesight and the development of some serious complications are not prevented by the use of glasses, injections and pills. Therefore, the number of blind people goes on increasing in spite of all possible medical aid.

WHY IS THIS SO? It is because the whole conception about the causes of errors of refraction is based on fallacies. When the sight begins to deteriorate, there must be some cause for it. And the cause is always an effort to see or strain. Glasses neutralize the effect but don't relieve the cause of trouble. So in some cases the cause continues increasing much by the use of glasses, hence the sight fails and some serious complications arise.

Almost all these cases of threatened blindness can be greatly benefited by eye education and mental relaxation. If the children and adults are taught about the proper use of eyes and relaxation, most of the defects of eyesight will fade away in a natural way.

Relief of Pain

When black is remembered perfectly, relief of pain always results. The skin may be pricked with a sharp instrument without causing discomfort. The lobe of the ear may be pinched between the nails of the thumb and first finger, and no pain will be felt. At the same time the sense of touch becomes more acute, the sense of taste, smell and hearing are also improved while the efficiency of the mind is increased. The ability to distinguish different temperatures is increased but one does not suffer from heat or cold.

A student was suffering from severe pain in the head and the eyes for many days. When he could palm and remember black he was completely relieved of pain.

In many cases of glaucoma not only the pain, but the tension which is often associated with the pain, has been completely relieved by palming.

A boy suffering from deafness began to hear well by the memory of black.

Why the memory of black should have such a good effect cannot be fully explained, but it is evident that the body must be less susceptible to disturbances of all kinds when the mind is under control, and when the mind is under control black can be remembered perfectly. That pain can be produced in any part of the body by the action of the mind is not a new observation; and if the mind can produce pain, it is not surprising that it should also be able to relieve pain and the conditions which produce it.

With a little training, anyone with good eyesight can be

taught to remember black properly with the eyes closed and covered, and with a little more training anyone can learn to do it with the eyes open. When one is suffering extreme pain, however, the control of the memory may be difficult and the assistance of someone who understands the method may be necessary.

The following case-reports have been written by the students of Dr. Agarwal.

1. Squint and its Cure

Sometimes children suffer much due to the wrong education received from parents or teachers who have some superstitions and thrust them upon the children under their influence.

When Jacqueline, a lady from Germany, was young, her father forced her to sit erect without any movement of the head or eyes while reading. She was told to keep the book at about 16 or 18 inches from the eyes as reading at a nearer distance was considered harmful. And she was advised not to read in dim light so that the eyes might not be spoiled. The result of these instructions is that she has suffered much. Her eyes have lost their symmetry and don't focus harmoniously. She gets double vision when she reads and when she tries to look to the side she gets a shooting pain and a severe headache. Her memory is so much affected that it takes her a long time to remember anything; so she has to read the same thing many a time and yet she is not sure that she has learnt it.

She consulted several eye specialists in Germany. All of them were of the opinion that the muscle of the left eye was weak; they could not help her in any way to relieve her eye troubles and her squint and she was thought a hopeless case.

Destiny fortunately brought her to India to visit Sri Aurobindo Ashram. Her neighbour at Parc, Mr. Ram Agarwal, casually told her about Dr. Agarwal at the School for Perfect Eyesight where his treatment was going on. Mr. Ram has come all the way from Bombay for his treatment and hearing all his story of threatened blindness she became curious to visit the School for Perfect Eyesight.

On the 30th July 1970 Jacqueline came here for consultation. Though she was a "hopeless case" Dr. Agarwal never gave up hope and listened to her patiently. In a few minutes' talk he grasped all her troubles and assured her that she would be all right within a few days.

She was then examined with the Ophthalmoscope and Retinoscope in the dark room. She was found absolutely normal. The perception of colour was also normal; even the field of vision was normal. She was then told to sit and read; she said that while moving the sight on the printed lines she got double vision by the time she reached the other end of the line. This was followed by shooting pain and headache. This was because in her earlier life she was taught to keep her face straight as if placed on the face-rest which was devised by a German doctor. These instructions made her unable to blink and shift the sight along with the head. This resulted in the development of strain and squint. The strain had led to all the discomforts which she was suffering.

Even the look in her eyes clearly showed that while seeing she strained. The expression of her left eye was at times completely blank. When she looked to her right or left, keeping her head stationary, one could easily see the squint in her eyes. While looking over her right shoulder the eye-ball of the left eye did not turn completely to the nasal side; similar was the case with her right eye though a little less. The German doctors had concluded that the muscle of her left eye was too weak; but they could not help her in any way.

After her examination, Dr. Agarwal made a treatment chart for her. She was then taught to discard all her old straining habits. She was also taught to blink and use the eyes properly while reading and writing. After this she was taken to the window for sun treatment, followed by eyewash and palming. This gave her relaxation. Then she was told to do long swing before bars and to read fine print in candle-light and good light alternately. This stimulated her eyes. Next was a game of ball; *i.e.*, throwing the ball from one palm to the other keeping the sight on the ball and blinking each time the ball was thrown; head and eyes should move together. This was the last exercise in her treatment chart.

The objective of this treatment was to relieve her of strain and strain only. First, if the strain could be removed, then only could she be benefited. To achieve this we gave her exercises of relaxation.

She practised this treatment for a week or so and the result is that she has improved greatly. She no more experiences shooting pain in her eyes. Her squint has completely disappeared. While reading there is no more double vision. She blinks often now and thus relaxes her eyes continually. Her expression of the eyes and face appears very beautiful and her memory too has improved.

2. Night Blindness which Came of Fear

Up till 2 years ago Srimati Sahu lived the normal life of a happy housewife with her 5 children. Then one of those unfortunate events that come to some people came in the form of dacoits (robbers), who attacked both her and her husband at their home in Orissa.

For the next 6 months she was unable to sleep at night, due to the thought that one night these people might return. Much as one is unable to sleep with a dripping tap, when one is constantly waiting for the next drip.

To pass away the long night hours Srimati Sahu took to reading. But so much reading under adverse conditions in time began to tell on her, and increasing difficulty in discerning the letters of the print was experienced. The condition deteriorated further and further until it was impossible to read even in daytime, and at night time complete blindness manifested itself after 5.30 p.m. To snatch a little bit of sleep the security of many people around her was needed, but these were sorry times for the family.

Relief was sought through the normal hospital methods. A well-known eye specialist at Cuttack gave a 4 month course of orthodox medical treatment. As no relief was obtained it seemed pointless to continue with the treatment. Another eye specialist of Cuttack was consulted, and a further treatment of 4 months undertaken, but with similar results.

At the beginning of 1970 an unseen light began to burn in the form of a suggestion from a friend, who said that they should go to have the Mother's February Darshan.

Bags were packed for the long trip to Pondicherry. During their stay the light burnt a little brighter when some one suggested to them that the School for Perfect Eyesight might be able to help her. At the School they found out that for any permanent relief a one-month's course of treatment would be needed, but, as duties at home prevented this, medicine and a chart were taken home for home treatment.

At home Srimati Sahu was unable to read even the largest letter of the chart, but with persistence of the treatment her daytime vision slowly improved, so that after 2 months the chart could be read right through. However, the night blindness still manifested itself with the onset of twilight.

Realizing that a longer course of treatment under the direct supervision of Dr. Agarwal might bring more rapid and furtheir relief, another visit was payed to Pondicherry for the April Darshan, after which she could stay for one month's treatment.

On testing her sight in ordinary daylight conditions we found that she could see and read quite well. However, on being taken into a dimly lit room there was no perception of things around her, even people standing in the room were not seen. By examining the internal parts of the eye with an optical instrument one could see nothing organically wrong, and as this showed that there must be a psychological cause the doctor said that some help could be given. Only time would show the extent of any improvement.

A course of treatment was duly begun, starting with sun treatment, when Srimati Sahu sat facing the morning sun with closed eyes gently swaying from side to side, so that the healing rays of the sun came through the eyelids, and entered the eye-ball to stimulate the blood vessels of the eye. This was followed by palming to relax the mind, long swing to relax the body nerves and muscles, concentration on a candle flame, playing with a ball to eliminate habits of staring. At the end she sat in a comfortable chair for one hour with ginger pads over the eyes to give the eyes a complete rest and allow them to rejuvenate.

After one week of this treatment there was a marked improvement, as she was now sleeping for 7 to 8 hours. In daytime when taken into a dimly lit room people around her could be seen, and the small letters on the chart could be read. Also it was possible to walk along the street during twilight hours, but, there always was a but, with the fall of night there was also a fall into night blindness once again.

This may sound strange to you, and equally it was strange to us, that she could see in a dim room during daytime, and yet could not see in a well illuminated room at night time. To find out the root cause of how this could be, Dr. Agarwal invited her and her husband to his room so that he could observe her actions during evening hours.

Arriving at the Doctor's house at 6.15 p.m. she could still see quite normally and even walked through the dim passage-way and up the stairs without any difficulty. The Doctor immediately put her to work preparing a fruit salad and doing other odd jobs.

At 7 p.m. when it was dark outside and we were relying completely on the electric light, my curiosity began to increase and I asked the husband, "But you have said she is unable to see in such light." He was also now aroused, and fired questions at her. "Can you see the milk?" he asked. Srimati Sahu began to stare to see if she could see things.

Once again she was under a strain with the result that the vision began to fail. In less than 5 minutes we could see that the night blindness was manifested once again as she now felt her way around the room. When they left the Doctor's house later in the evening she had to be led down the stairs and along the street.

The Doctor was now able to conclude that what brought the blindness on was the firing of questions at her, and so instructed the husband and everyone else that this was not to be done in future. Rather she should be given something to do to occupy her mind, thus stopping any tendency to stare.

Under the one month course of treatment her night vision

still continued to improve. Three weeks after commencing the vision was in such a good state that it was possible to go to the cinema, after which she could walk back to the guest house along the dark streets.

The light which had first been lit by the friend's suggestion 5 months ago was now burning with a steady flame. And Srimati Sahu was able to return to her family to lead a normal happy life.

In early August, 2 months after having finished our treatment we received a letter from Orissa. Srimati Sahu was still well and happy, there being no relapse into the troubles of bygone days.

This case very pointedly shows that the orthodox method of tablets, injections, glasses, etc., is not always the answer to psychological problems. But rather one may show outstanding improvement when following natural means of treatment.

3. A Case of Glaucoma

The eyes and the mind are closely associated. The strain of one affects the other. And if the mind is under a strain due to some physical discomfort and at that time if one makes an effort to read or strain to see distant objects there is usually a rapid fall in one's eyesight. The following case is a good illustration of this fact.

A case of threatened blindness, a scientist working in Regional Research Laboratory, Bhubaneshwar, had been suffering from eye-trouble since February 70. He lost much of his vision because he strained to see distant objects under unfavourable conditions diagnosed as Gastritis. Further when he was examined in Sarojini Devi Eye Hospital, Doctors declared the that patient was suffering from low tension glaucoma and was given 200 tablets and 36 injections but all in vain. Moreover, they did not give any definite hope of improvement by means of medicines or operation.

He was then examined by us thoroughly. He had been using glasses for 12 years but for last few months even with glasses the distant vision was blurred and the near vision beginning to fail. His vision was recorded 10/100 without or with glasses, he developed colour blindness and night blindness. Also frequent reading was followed by shooting pain. Tension was normal when examined with two fingers.

Other interesting observations about him were: he took a long time for accommodation to see at near point as well as for distance. It took him more than a minute or two to read the big print. Lines of smaller print seemed to him like thick black lines. Print which was not clear from a normal distance, usually caused pain when brought nearer for reading. The colour, size, and form of the letters or objects regarded altered greatly for him.

It is important to note this fact clearly that the vision is a process of mental interpretation. The picture which the mind sees is not the impression on the retina but the mental interpretation or the imagination of it. When the vision is imperfect, the interpretation or the imagination also becomes imperfect and the mind adds imperfections to the imperfect retinal images.

On this basis the treatment of the patient began. It was firstly based on swinging and correction of the position of the lids, after the usual exercises of Sun treatment and Palming. He was taught to develop control over his imagination or the power of interpretation by the various exercises of central fixation, memory and imagination. As soon as the patient learnt to relax the mind and imagine something according to reality the conditions which had led to a distortion and imperfection of images began to subside. In fact, mental relaxation is the key to curing most of the eye troubles.

The exercises of mental relaxation proved marvellously successful. The improvement in his case is indisputable. Symptoms of colour blindness and night blindness have almost faded and he can see fairly well at a distance. He feels comfortable in moving about at night without glasses. He is no more afraid of the threatened blindness. He enjoys nature and its beauty like a normal person.

Along with the improvement in his eyesight there has been also some remarkable improvement in his general physical condition. His trouble of Gastritis has subsided. He feels free from suffering, worry and anxiety. His ability to do things has greatly increased. The patient takes a lot of interest in doing the exercises of Eye Education and Mental Relaxation in the calm atmosphere of the School for Perfect Eyesight.

4. A Case of High Compound Myopia

The fast increase in the power of glasses and the development of some serious complications in some myopic patients leads them towards blindness and all the methods of treatment with the orthodox medical practitioners fail to prevent this deterioration. In this state of utter hopelessness, with his sight rapidly getting worse, Ram heard about Dr. Agarwal through a friend who is a regular reader of Mother India, a monthly journal of the Sri Aurobindo Ashram, in which articles on eye education, written by Dr. Agarwal are regularly appearing. The unusualness of his methods and the wonderful cures achieved, were a promise to Ram and he came all the way from

Bombay to undergo a course of treatment at the School for Perfect Eyesight.

His was a case of high compound myopia coupled with alternate divergent squint. In spite of the correction with glasses the vision was poor and his squint still persisted. He was using glasses of -13 with a cylinder of -3. When he was five years old, he had started using glasses of -1. From then onwards the power had increased until it had reached the present number.

Reading with these glasses caused such a great strain that he had to discontinue his studies, a few weeks before the exams. The tension of preparing for the test had increased his eye strain to an unbearable extent and he was facing a gloomy future. This mental strain and eye strain is the cause of such a fast deterioration in eyesight.

Out in the bright sunlight Ram experienced splitting headaches. He just could not venture out without very dark sun glasses. When he looked up at heights he would go temporarily blind due to appearance of a dark cloud. Often floating specks also appeared before his eyes. Observations showed that he found reading without glasses more comfortable.

Dr. Agarwal examined his eyes in the dark-room with the ophthalmoscope and found the condition of the retina in an unhealthy state but had some hope of improvement as the patient had flashes of improved vision at times.

The treatment chart included blinking education, sun treatment, palming, swinging and central fixation and reading fine print in good light and candle light. His diet was modified to include more greens and fruits. At times an enema was also given to relieve him from gas trouble.

After about a fortnight Ram expressed a cheerful outlook, he was moving about without glasses, his reading became quite convenient. The gloomy future due to threatened blindness vanished from his mind for ever. It is hoped that Ram will be able to go about his work once again with relaxed eyes and mind. After a short treatment he expressed his experience in the following letter:

"Prior to the treatment at the School for Perfect Eyesight I visualised a very dark future as my eyesight then deteriorated gradually. But now after I have started the School's treatment I feel that there is hope for me and that I have all possibilities of improvement. My heart is now full of hope and I anxiously look forward to the bright future.

There has been a gradual improvement. All the headaches and the strain in the eyes have disappeared. My sight too shows a steady progress. This is indicated by the fact that previously I could see the top letter C at only 5 ft. without my glasses, but today I noticed that the same letter is now visible from 16 ft."

5. A Story from the Clinic

Raju was a bright and intelligent lad, always topping the class. The final exams were a month ahead. Raju was hoping to get a first class and was studying hard for it.

All went well until a week before the test. Raju began to have splitting headaches. He just could not concentrate. An hour's study would make his head and eyes pain. If one hour was so unbearable, what about the hours of study that lay ahead.

His aunt, who was on a visit with his people, heard about poor Raju from his parents. She smiled and said she would put things right. Now this wise lady had been following Dr.

Bates' system of eye care, and has maintained her sight in a perfect state.

She stepped into Raju's study to find her nephew swallowing his third aspirin. She walked up to his desk. The dazzling light of the high power table lamp fell on the open pages of a book.

"Cause One of your headache," she said. "This light creates a glare which hurts your eyes. Switch off the light and read in the soft light of a candle." Her nephew did so.

"Cause Two of your discomfort," went on the aunt, "Are you an old man that you should hold your book at such a distance? Hold it closer and your eyes will not tire.

"Cause Three. You do not rest your eyes. Blink at the end of each line and you can study with ease for longer hours.

"As a parting gift, here is a book of Fine Print which you should read once every day to keep your sight in perfect order till a ripe old age. Now goodbye and the best of luck!"

The exams were over and the results were out. It was a proud Raju who bagged the first prize. "It's all thanks to aunty and her instructions", smiled the happy boy.

Optician and the Doctor

Q: What is God?
A: God is Perfection.

Q: Dr. J. does not believe in God.
A: But he believes in perfection of man and his conception is quite right within his own spheres. Everyone has a different conception of God so long as he does not realise Him in himself.

Q: We had a long discussion about the existence of God.

A: The existence of God cannot be known by discussions, it can be known only by realisation. One can speak as much in favour as against.

Q: *What is perfection?*
A: Do you lose your temper sometime or get depressed? "Yes."
It means loss of mental control, an imperfection. Perfect mental control under all conditions of life is an aspect of perfection. Such a perfection is possible by Integral Yoga, by the realisation of God in oneself and in others.

Q: *Why did you leave your practice and settle here in the Ashram?*
A: Such was the call in me and this has greatly benefited myself as well as my sons.

Q: *Is it really true that defective eyesight can be improved without glasses?*
A: Almost all the Ophthalmologists of the world believe that there is neither prevention nor cure for the errors of refraction. Don't you believe then that Ophthalmic Science is yet in a very imperfect stage?
"Yes".
Dr. W. H. Bates of America realised this very early in his practice; so through a series of experiments and observations he found the fallacies of the orthodox practitioners and proved by experiments and clinical treatment that defective eyesight could be improved without glasses by eye education and mental relaxation.

Q: *My wife suffers from a severe headache after driving. Eye*

Specialists find no fault with her general condition.
A: Yet there is some fault otherwise why should she suffer?

Q: Can you cure her?
A: Yes, in three days.

Q: Can you show me some cases who have been benefited by your methods of eye education?
A: Here are cases of myopia, hypermetropia, presbyopia and early cataract. You may talk to them and satisfy yourself.

Q: Yes, I am convinced. Is there any book on this subject?
A: Here are *Mind and Vision, Better Sight, Care of Eyes.* Would you like to put these books in your optical shop.
"No, Doctor; this will go against our profession, but I will bring my wife for treatment."

Q: You recommend fine print reading, but will it not cause strain?
A: Dr. Bates has made many remarkable discoveries relative to the prevention and cure of imperfect sight without the aid of glasses. The most remarkable discovery is this:
Fine Print is a Benefit to the Eye. Large Print is a Menace.
Fine print cannot be read well unless the eyes are relaxed. Reading fine print in good light and in candle light alternately is extremely beneficial to prevent and cure all sorts of eye defects. Any one can test this truth and fact.

Q: What is the aim of this School for Perfect Eyesight?
A: It trains people how to get rid of eye troubles. It will create doctors of new thought and new knowledge to help the suffering humanity.

It is time that some doctors should carefully study Dr. Bates' works and repeat his experiments if necessary. If one discards his works without proper study, then surely the person is not a true scientist, he is like a religionist who believes in particular dogmas.

Q: One more question: can God be seen?
A: Yes, but not with these external eyes; for that, one has to develop the inner eye or the divine eye.

The Divine Eye

Q: What do you mean by the divine eye or divine vision?
A: You see so many things in the world. How?
"By these external eyes."
And in dream also you see so many things, how?
"Don't know."
Through the mental eye. But God's Shakti is hidden in everything, in stone, in plant, in animal, in man; this Shakti is visible through the divine eye. When the divine eye is developed, the consciousness of man is changed.
"Where is the seat of the divine eye?"
Between the eyebrows.

Q: Can the system of eye education help the development of the divine eye or inner eye?
A: Eye education means mental relaxation. When the mind is at rest and has relaxation, then it is easy for the higher forces to descend so as to develop the inner eye.

Q: What relaxation exercises will be most helpful?
A: Some patients have reported that while doing palming

and concentration on candle flame they had experiences of the descent of Peace and Light and Joy and Force.

Q: Normal vision means perfect relaxation of the mind and eyes. Do you mean then that every person with the normal eye can develop the divine eye?

A: If there is a sincere aspiration for the Divine.

Q: What do you mean by a change of consciousness which comes by the development of the divine eye?

A: I answer this question through a dialogue:

King Aswapathy and Rajguru

King: What is a change of consciousness?

Rajguru: O King, develop the divine eye so as to become conscious of thy soul and God. You will see His presence in everyone, you will feel one with others. Ego will fade away.

King: How to develop the divine eye?

Rajguru: By Yoga.

King: What is Yoga?

Rajguru:

> United with Him,
> Divine within,
>   Yoga it is.

> Surrender to Him,
> Work for Him,
>   Yoga it is.

Love for Him,
Desire nothing,
Yoga it is.

The King does Yoga. He surrenders to his Guru. He concentrates in his heart. There he sees fire. In the heart's fire the old physical consciousness is dissolved. The soul is born. Her name is Savitri.

The consciousness of the King has changed. He experiences the presence of the Divine Mother in his heart and feels her Shakti in his works. He gets inspirations. He is full of love and feels one with others. His aim of life is to bring a change in the consciousness of the world. He sings a song in joy and Ananda:

Mother Divine,
Sun of the Heaven,
Sea of Ananda,
I pray to Thee.

Mother Divine,
Love of my heart,
Beauty of my eyes,
I offer to Thee.

Mother Divine,
Force of the life,
Light of the mind,
I work for Thee.

Savitri, the soul of King Aswapathy, is on the mountain of Truth, she meets a Sannyasi:

Sannyasi: O Virgin, where are you going?

Savitri: I go to meet the Supreme. One day I will return with His Shakti and change the world.

Sannyasi: This is impossible. This ignorant world cannot be changed. Come with me to Nirvana.

The Divine Sage **Narad** appears. Narayana, Narayana.

Narad: O Sannyasi, I have three mangoes, tell me their condition.

Sannyasi: This is quite unripe.

This is about to be ripe.

This is perfectly ripe.

Narad: All the three mangoes are of the same tree. The ripe mango was unripe at one time. Like the ripe mango the world will become ripe one day. It will be full of peace, joy and Ananda. God's Shakti Supramental is working in it. The consciousness of the world will be changed.

How Does Savitri Bring a Change?

Savitri is the soul, the divine flame in the heart, Savitri is the light in the mind, Savitri is the force of life, Savitri is the peace of the body. When Savitri grows up, she goes to the Supreme to bring His light, His Power, His Love and Ananda. She meets Satyavan and surrenders to Him. With his help she transforms the nature and the body. She manifests Beauty, Harmony, Love and Ananda and divine life.

Note: Read this passage again and again with Central Fixation, each word regarded appearing darker.

SYNTHESIS

Our aim is to create new type of doctors to relieve the sufferings of the humanity and to manifest health and happiness and perfect eyesight. They will be guided by their intuition and their knowledge will be based on the synthesis of all the systems of medicine.

Along with the evolution of man's intelligence, medicine has also evolved. At first the means of evolution were sense faculties and intuition and that discovery of medicine was called Ayurveda or Indian Medicine. Then the intellect discovered various diagnostic intruments, such as microscope, X'rays, Ophthalmoscope, etc., since the knowledge through sense perception was found insufficient by the rational mind; this discovery of medicine was called Allopathy or Modern Medicine. Hahnemann observed that the life-force was affected in sickness and he evolved Homeopathy. Bates noted that the mind was under a great strain in most of the eye troubles and physical ailments, and he developed relaxation methods. Thus each system covers a part of the complex medicine and attempts to bring out its highest possibilities. A synthesis of all of them largely conceived and applied will result in the integral system of medicine. But they are so disparate in their tendencies that we do not easily find how we can arrive at their right union. An undiscriminating combination will create confusion. The synthesis we propose must seize some central principles common to all which will include and utilize in the right place and proportion their particular principles. The source of life is **LIFE ENERGY** which pervades in the universe and descends from the Unknown summit. Its flow in the organ or organs of the body is disturbed by strain due to any reason. In the case of visual defects the strain immediately appears when there is an effort to see. The normal eye functioning normally never makes an effort to see, it functions like other sense organs without any effort on its part. So when there is an effort to see the nerves of the eye and mind are under strain. To relieve this strain a triune process is to be adopted. This process is based on three principles:—

1. Elimination:— Elimination of toxic matter and bad habits and wrong use of the organ.

2. Stimulation:— Stimulation of the vitality of the organ by certain methods.

3. Relaxation of the mind and nerves by relaxation exercises.

We will detail this triune process later on. It is a fact that every system of medicine has developed a part of this triune process and a harmonious combination of all of them will yield wonderful results to root out the sufferings of the humanity and man will enjoy perfect eyesight. Hence to achieve great success the integral knowledge of medicine is essential in its basic principles, but the proper sense of integration and efficiency will develop in a physician more and more by the evolution of the Spirit in him.

This integral knowledge in Ophthalmic Science is being taught to the students of the School for Perfect Eyesight, Sri Aurobindo Ashram, Pondicherry through a four year course.

This spiritualised doctor of the future will prove to be a physician *par excellence*, integrating all the systems of medicine harmoniously. In the diagnosis and treatment of patients he will be mainly guided by his intuition though he may also make use of modern scientific instruments to express the phenomena in scientific terms. His methods of treatment will be simple and harmless and will bring quick recovery, even in many so-called hopeless cases. His very presence will radiate peace and healing force and his patient will be conscious of him as a saviour.

A lady patient aged thirty-five had developed insomnia and total nightblindness. The doctors of Orissa failed to give her any relief. This patient was treated through the triune process and was completely cured in a month's time. A boy whose eyesight had failed for distance and near gained normal vision in about two weeks' time. Almost all cases developing defective vision or blindness can be greatly benefited by the integral system of medicine though Dr. Bates system of relaxation plays a very important part in the treatment. It is such a thing that should be taught to our students in the medical institutions. The old rut ought to be replaced by the integral system of medicine.

Perfection in Eyesight

Our homage to Sri Aurobindo and the Divine Mother who have brought down the Supramental Power on the earth to bring a change in the consciousness of man for the flowering of life. Due to the pressure of that Light man is now more open to accept new truths and ideas. There are some enlightened doctors in the medical profession who are not satisfied with the old routine of treatment due to its detrimental effects and feel the need to do some real good to humanity; to such persons of goodwill the following points are exposed for consideration:

1. It is a fact that glasses help many to relieve their discomforts of the head and eyes and enable people to see well at a distance and near, and their use in many cases is imperative. But this is also true that glasses do not check further deterioration and the number of glasses goes on increasing. Often

glasses become an added torture to increase the pain and suffering and loss of eyesight. The problem of fast deterioration in eyesight and the increase of blind people amongst the educated class has become quite serious in the present time in spite of all possible medical aid and we should feel ashamed for this helplessness.

2. Process of seeing is mostly done in the brain; our vision is mind's interpretation of the retinal images. Relaxation of mind helps to see well while mental strain causes defective vision. The old writers on Ophthalmology did not consider that the mental strain could play an important part in the formation of errors of refraction and other diseases of the eye, hence they isolated the eye while determining the cause and treatment of visual defects and retinal disorders. This has led to our failure.

3. The incurability of errors of refraction is based on the theory that the eye changes its focus for vision at different distances by altering the curvature of the lens. Dr. W. H. Bates M.D., an American Scientist and Ophthalmologist, when found himself incapable to prevent myopia and other errors of refraction, felt that there must be something wrong in the presumption of this theory. So he performed many experiments to determine the facts about accommodation and errors of refraction. He has made many remarkable discoveries:

(a) In accommodation the eye adjusts its focus like a camera by a change in the length of the organ, and this alteration is brought about by the action of external eye muscles called Oblique muscles.

(b) Myopia is not caused by reading but by a strain to see distant objects. Strain at the near point causes hypermetropia.

(c) Reading fine print is extremely beneficial to the eyes.

(d) By eye education and mental relaxation almost all cases of defective vision can be cured partially or completely.

(e) Myopia can be easily prevented in schools by reading the Snellen Eye Testing Chart daily with gentle blinking and palming.

Why have the Ophthalmologists Failed to Prevent Visual Defects? It is because theories of about two hundred years back have been taken as facts and this has served to obscure the truth and to stop further investigation. When visual defects cannot be prevented even, this is an indication of some great imperfection in the science. However, in the light of truth the problem of loss of eyesight and increased blindness is simple and the solution is quite easy and practical. It has been proved in thousands of cases that errors of refraction are easily preventable and curable by the methods of Relax and See and the cases of threatened blindness due to glaucoma, optic atrophy, retinitis pigmentosa, macular degeneration and retinitis etc., can be greatly benefited. Here I mention two cases as an illustration:

Dr. R. K. Puri of Pondicherry Medical College states the condition of his son. "My son, Rakesh, was complaining of watering and fatigue in the eyes specially while reading. The doctor in charge of the eye department examined the boy under atropine and prescribed glasses of +1.5 for the right eye and +2.5 for the left eye. By these glasses watering did not stop and a sort of depression and irritation appeared in the temperament of the boy. Why such a thing happened suddenly, we could not understand though the boy had improved his vision with glasses. We took the boy to the School for Perfect Eyesight. When the treatment started glasses were discarded. This itself greatly relieved the boy and he felt very happy. At the end of the treatment his sight was again tested and it was a surprise to us that the boy was having normal sight both for distance and near and all his watering and strain vanished in three days and we found his temperament also changed for good."

Another remarkable case of an American girl scholar wearing glasses of -7.0 who learnt the art of seeing and gained almost normal sight in a few days. As she puts it: "I can now read almost the whole chart without the lenses. I can also read a book at one foot distance, which was not possible before."

Hints for the Prevention and Cure of Visual Defects:

1. Some ophthalmologists of goodwill may be appointed by the Government to repeat the experiments of Dr. Bates. For practical study they may be sent to the School for Perfect Eyesight.

2. When truth is discovered scientifically, it ought to be introduced in the medical curriculum of medical colleges.

3. For successful working it will be necessary to establish an International Institute of Ophthalmology where the teaching should be based on the synthesis of all the systems of medicine. Such a synthesis I have already explained in my books. A diploma Course of 4 years in Ophthalmic Science may be introduced in this institution. Students joining this institution need not go to complete M.B., B.S. For medical graduates one year training will be sufficient. Students qualifying from this institution will prove very successful in life to relieve the sufferings of humanity.

4. The scheme to prevent visual defects may be soon started in the schools.

5. Public may be educated about the simple methods of Relax and See through books, pamphlets, periodicals and movies.

If the work is sincerely adopted without prejudice and perversity, then the Indian Ophthalmologists will have an important and honourable place in the world, their service will be highly appreciated.

We aim to create a new type of doctor who will bring perfection in eyesight. His knowledge will be based on the synthesis. He will be more concerned with the health than with the pathology. To achieve this aim the School provides a course in Ophthalmic Science.

CHAPTER XII

LETTERS OF SRI AUROBINDO

(*This is the opening instalment of Dr. R. S. Agarwal's questions and Sri Aurobindo's answers. Dr. Agarwal made his first pilgrimage to Pondicherry on July 2, 1934. While in the Ashram he used to visit a Maharaja, a non-Ashramite, who was an exile from the then British India. In the Maharaja's company he found his mind turning hostile to the Mother. So he wanted to run away from the Ashram after a few days. His inner struggle was reaching a climax when he met an old sadhika, Gopiben, who tried to help him see the Ashram life correctly. One day, after a talk with her, he returned to his room, fell asleep and felt a powerful light penetrating his chest. This was the beginning of a series of spiritual experiences and marked a revolution in his life. All the correspondence we are publishing was carried on during his short visits to the Ashram. Dr. Agarwal has been a permanent resident of the Ashram since 1955 and runs there the School for Perfect Eyesight.* Mother India.)

On Eyesight without Glasses

Self: At present I have my eye-clinic at Bulandshar. I go to Delhi to work twice a week. I now find that there is a better field at Delhi for my profession. So I propose to move wholly over to Delhi in the month of October. But first I must know what you think about it. I need your permission and protection above all. For the shifting of the clinic to the capital is a matter of great responsibility.

SRI AUROBINDO: It seems to me that Delhi is clearly indicated — so you can start your work there in October.

7-7-1934

Self: You have given me your Blessings to start the Eye-hospital at Delhi. Sometimes I get dejected owing to my poor financial condition; but at once you appear before me and, changing into Lord Krishna, you say, "Why do you fear about anything? I have already arranged everything for you. Simply proceed and begin the work there. It is I who am to take care and not you." Is this really an inner voice or an imagination?

SRI AUROBINDO: No, it is not an imagination.

8-7-1934

Self: The Mother might be using glasses for reading. Would she like to try my treatment?

SRI AUROBINDO: The Mother has seen that these methods are perfectly effective, but she cannot follow a treatment because she has no time. Her sight is variable: when she can rest and concentrate a little and do what is necessary, she can read without glasses.

8-7-1934

Self: I propose three names to the Mother to select from for my Delhi hospital.

(1) *Eye sanatorium*

(2) *Dr. Agarwal's Eye Institute*

(3) *Ram Eye Charitable Hospital.*

The Mother put a cross at the second proposal and wrote below:

"A name for Agarwal's institution"

14-7-1934

SRI AUROBINDO: Keep a complete trust and work. You have a sufficient openness in you in your work for the Power to act; but a complete faith and courage are needed.

Our blessings are with you.

6-10-1934

SRI AUROBINDO: I am in receipt of two letters from you. We are glad to hear that the opening ceremony (of the Delhi hospital) passed off well.

Certainly, if it is helpful for you to take students, then you can do so. If the student from Patna comes, you can keep him or anyone else who offers and seems to have capacity for the work.

Whatever difficulties occur, call down the help and force of the Divine and go through. But keep in the midst of your work a part of your mind turned towards them[1] and open to receive the force of the Mother.

28-10-1934

SRI AUROBINDO: We are glad to hear that the hospital work was successful in October. It is sure to expand, keeping the Force behind you, and become more successful. That is the condition of success always, faith, courage, openness to the Force.

10-11-1934

Self: During my lectures, people ask me this question: "In Yoga, while concentrating on a picture or idol one should not blink. Why then do you advise us to blink always?" I used to think they

----
[1] Uncertain reading (Editor.)

were wrong in raising this question. But now I see the truth of that side. Blinking automatically stops when one is deeply concentrated on an outer image. For one becomes almost blind to the external environment. I want to know if such non-blinking will cause strain and defective eyesight.

SRI AUROBINDO: It is partly true. But the Yogins who practise *trāṭak* put a force in the eyes which counteracts the effects of the non-blinking.

6-4-1935

Self: You wrote to me that you had kept me under your protection. Till recently I was unable to understand the working of the protection. Now its action becomes visible in my hospital work. I find that every patient is under its influence: it is especially marked when his disease is serious or efficient treatment is not offered to him by my assistants; then it is just astonishing to watch how the Mother makes the patient all right. When I am much interested in a particular case, because of the complexities of the symptoms, I invoke the Mother's help. I feel that her Force does come down. What do you say about all this?

SRI AUROBINDO: Yes, it is true. That is quite the right way.

6-4-1935

SRI AUROBINDO: We are very glad to learn of your success in Nepal; it shall be a great help to you in your work. If they ask you in May, you should certainly accept the offer . I trust that now you are there the hospital work will pick up again and go on with more activity and success.

Keep yourself open by steady sadhana, bhakti and self-offering. Our blessings and protection are with you.

31-12-1935

About Sadhana

*Q: When in Pondicherry I feel your presence most of the time.
But when I am on my way back to Delhi, even on reaching Madras
it fades away. Why is that so? How could I preserve it everywhere.*

SRI AUROBINDO: It is easier to feel the presence in the
atmosphere of the Ashram than outside it. But that is only an
initial difficulty which one can overcome by a steadiness in the
call and a constant opening of oneself to the influence.

*Q: A gentleman from Kashmir was staying in a hotel at Madras.
He could read anything with the help of one of his fingers while his
eyes were completely bandaged. I went to see him simply to gain
some knowledge for the treatment of the blind. He said, "All this is
due to improvement in the inner vision. If you want to improve
your inner vision, just try this: place a lighted candle in front and
gaze at the bright colour of the flame as long as you can. When
you feel any strain close the eyes and imagine as if it is quite dark
before the eyes or imagine some interesting or pleasant object.
This is better practised at bed-time."*

*I tried it for the first time at Bangalore just before going to bed.
Well, during the sleep some fearful object appeared before me. I
got frightened and remembered Lord Krishna. The object soon
vanished. After sometime another came, and that too disappeared
when I thought of Lord Krishna. Then I understood that all that
was due to my gazing on the flame. So I decided not to practise it
or, if at all, only at Pondicherry.*

*Well, was that really due to the gazing at the flame? Should
I attempt it here?*

SRI AUROBINDO: This gazing on a flame or on a bright
spot is the traditional means used by many Yogins for concen-

tration or for awakening of the inner consciousness and vision. You seem to have gone by this gazing into a kind of surface (not deep) trance, which is indeed one of its first results and begun to see things probably on the vital plane. I do not know what were the "dreadful objects" you saw, but that dreadfulness is the character of many things first seen on that plane, especially when crossing its threshold by such means. You should not employ them, I think, for they are quite unnecessary and, besides, they may lead to a passive concentration in which one is open to all sorts of things and cannot choose the right ones.

Q: On the 4th August, at Madras, I felt as if there was a wooden temple. The light was passing out through its holes. When the door came in front of me, I saw Lord Krishna standing by the side of a cow. Is that all from an inner vision?

SRI AUROBINDO: You say you felt — it was only an impression or you *saw* in a mental vision or other image? If the latter it was the inner vision — if only a feeling, then the vision was deep within *veiled* by the mind and what you got was only an impression of it thrown upon the mind.

Q: On the 5th August, at Madras, while offering prayers I felt myself sitting under the trees and offering prayers to Lord Krishna. What does it mean?

SRI AUROBINDO: It was a mental experience — you put yourself in contact with Krishna and it took that form in your mind.

Q: At about 5 p.m. yesterday I was taking some physical exercise. In the course of it I experienced as if you were doing the exercise for me! That happened only for a short while and yet seemed so delightful. But when I tried to keep up with that imagination continuously, it vanished. I am at a loss to understand what it meant.

SRI AUROBINDO: It was not an imagination, but an experience. When such an experience occurs, the attempt to take hold of it mentally and continue it may on the contrary interrupt it. It is best to let it continue of itself — if it ceases, it is likely to recur.

Q: This morning while sitting on my terrace I was offering my prayers to God. All on a sudden I got into this vision:

An earthen pot black in colour surged up before me. Flames were coming out of it. They went on increasing and with them some black things were coming out in large numbers. These things assembled on a wall and seemed to be some beings. Then the flames went on decreasing. The black things lessened. Later on all the flames vanished and there remained no black things within them. The final appearance of the flames was reddish golden yellow free from any impurity. Afterwards the pot burst into pieces and Lord Krishna and Radha appeared. The light seemed to be very intense around them:

My own explanation of the vision:

The earthen pot was my body. The black things the weaknesses and the hostile forces. The fire was the Divine's love. Lord Krishna represented the Divine and Radha the Mother.

SRI AUROBINDO: Your explanation is fairly correct. But the pot was not the body, it was the old physical consciousness, and the flame was the flame of purification, Agni Pavaka. The reddish golden yellow colour indicates the flame of the Truth in the physical.

Q: After the above experience the vision changed. Now I was talking with the Mother just as I had done yesterday (during my interview). The whole arrangement of her room was the same. At a distance from this room I noticed a temple of Goddess Durga in which there appeared many lights before the feet of the Goddess. These lights were sometimes four, sometimes one, sometimes many in number. The single light was very very white, and in size bigger than all the others.

SRI AUROBINDO: The lights are the Mother's Powers — many in number. The white light is her own characteristic power, that of the Divine Consciousness in its essence — the four are probably those of her four principal powers described in the book "The Mother."

What you see is a symbolic image of the Mother in the various actions of her Powers, one, fourfold and manifold.

Q: I have egoistic desires and passions. I want them to be removed totally from me. What should be done for that?

SRI AUROBINDO: It is a matter of self-discipline and opening of the being to the Divine.

Q: I want to start every action of mine after knowing the Divine Will. But how to find out the Divine Will?

SRI AUROBINDO: It needs a quiet mind — in the quiet mind turned towards the Divine, the initiation comes of the Divine Will and the right way to do it.

Q: When in Pondicherry, I sometimes remember my children (residing in Delhi) and feel a little sorry. But I am soon awakened to the truth that there is nothing in the world to love except the Divine. This struggle goes on. How to be relieved of it?

SRI AUROBINDO: It is as the love of the Divine grows that the other things cease to trouble the mind.

Q: Today when I was taking my food I noticed for a moment that Lord Krishna was taking it with my spoon. I had a smile from him and then the figure disappeared.

SRI AUROBINDO: That is an experience sadhaks often have — that it is the Divine who is taking the meal.

Q: While sitting for meditation I see the figure of the Divine at two different places. One on the forehead and the other somewhere in the mind. It seems easier to hold the image for sometime in the first than in the second place.

SRI AUROBINDO: There is a centre of consciousness (chakra) in the forehead which is among other things the direct centre of inner vision — that is why it is easier to hold the image there. The other must be a mental image and can be held long only if the mind is very still.

Q: Today during prayer-time I felt as if there was a mountain beyond a sea. The saints were going to the mountain. They invited me to join them. But I said, "I have been sent here (on the earth) by the Divine to perform certain duties; hence it is not the time for me to accompany you." Then a vague image of Lord Krishna appeared before me and approved of my statement. What does all this indicate?

SRI AUROBINDO: It indicates probably that the possibility of a spiritual realisation (the mountain) beyond life (the sea) such as the Sanyasins seek was put before you. Your refusal saying that you had a work to do for the Divine in the world and could not leave it and your answer was approved by the Divine.

Q: Yesterday evening, an Ashramite and I had a talk about snakes. The same night during my sleep I saw a big snake coming out of a basket kept in a cupboard. Seeing the snake I got very frightened, got up from the bed and went to my neighbour Venkat-raman. He at once came to my room. Then I read a book of the teachings of Sri Ramakrishna. After a time, I went to sleep again, placing your photograph under my pillow. Then there was no dreadful dream and I slept well.

What was that nightmare due to? Kindly keep me under your protection so that such terrifying figures may not appear before me.

SRI AUROBINDO: It must have been merely because you talked of snakes — it created an impression in the mind which came up from the subconscient in sleep. Fear of things seen in sleep or vision should be altogether dismissed — the attitude taken should be that the divine protection is with you and these things cannot harm you.

Q: I kept the photos of the Mother and yourself in front of me and then began to meditate. Through them I prayed to you to grant me happiness while I was here, and also for some experi-ences as I could not have any for a long time. Afterwards I felt the reflection of your photo in my heart. Later I felt as if there was no body except the head. In the place of my body there appeared a house where Lord Krishna as a boy was playing on a flute, sitting in a cradle, His mother and some other persons were moving the cradle forward and backward. I experienced happiness.

After the meditation I went to take my meal. On the way I felt the presence sometimes of yourself and sometimes of Lord Krishna.

SRI AUROBINDO: All these are experiences attended by mental images. It is your aspiration that awakes these forms and brings an answer in this kind of experiences which are preparing your consciousness for a more lasting and profound kind about which you yourself will not have any questioning — for they will be too vivid and real for that.

Your experience about the head and body would seem to indicate that the natural centre for your sadhana is in the heart and not in the head. If it is so, it is in the heart-centre (not the physical heart, but the cardiac centre in the middle of the chest) that you must concentrate, for there will be the focus of your experiences.

Q: X asks me to write you this for herself: "I feel the Mother's presence in my heart. I have not so much devotion that I can get an opportunity to see you. I pray for your blessings for the short-comings of my worldly life."

SRI AUROBINDO: Convey to her our blessings. Devotion and all else will develop if she makes the presence she feels the centre of her life, referring and offering all to it.

Q: During my evening prayer your image surged up before me and thus I talked with it: "I do not want anything except your presence within me." Kindly explain.

SRI AUROBINDO: It is something that took place in the mind — it can hardly be called an experience.

Q: Mother, I pray to you to arrange for Sri Aurobindo's Darshan once before I go from here. I understand it is against the rule. But I do feel that for a bhakta there is no rule.

SRI AUROBINDO: I am afraid it is impossible. No separate personal darshan can be given at this stage — it is not a rule, it is a necessity for the work that Sri Aurobindo is doing.

Q: I do not yet know if I am on the path of the true conscious-ness. I pray to you for some directions that may take me easily to the Truth.

SRI AUROBINDO: What has developed in you is a power of

true inner vision — this will help you to enter through it into touch with the Divine; you have only to let it develop. Two other things have to develop — the feeling of the Divine Presence and Power and inspiration behind your actions, and the inner contact with myself and with the Mother. Aspire with faith and sincerity and these will come. I do not wish to give any more precise instructions until I see what happens in you during your stay here — for although the path is common to all, each man has his own way of following it.

Q: Last evening I had the vision that you were standing in front of me. I requested you, "Kindly take me to the Divine." You asked me to follow you; and then you escorted me to a mountain. We climbed on and on till we attained a very high peak where the temple of Mother Durga was located. I bowed and got her blessings. Afterwards we ascended farther on where Lord Krishna was. Making my pranams I received his blessings. Then I prayed to the Lord, "Please grant me peace and wisdom." He replied, "These things you can have from Sri Aurobindo." Later we returned home.

SRI AUROBINDO: It is a mental vision, the images being supplied by the mind. The mountain always represents the ascending hill of existence with the Divine to be reached on the summit. In your vision you got the contact with the Divine and were told to seek peace and knowledge from me.

Q: Then I felt as if the Mother had been standing on the terrace silently, with closed eyes, and all the sadhaks standing below. It was evening.

SRI AUROBINDO: That again is a mental vision. These mental visions are meant to bring in the mind the influence of the things they represent — here the effect of the Mother's meditation and blessing in the evening.

Q: Is there any probability of my encountering the hostile forces? If so, how to face them?

SRI AUROBINDO: It is better not to trouble about the hostile forces. Keep your aspiration living and sincere and call in the Divine in each thing and each moment for support and all that you feel or need and keep yourself open to us. That is the easiest way to the Divine. If you begin to concern yourself with the hostile forces, you will only make the path difficult and troublesome.

Q: Today before taking my lunch I remembered you, but you did not appear before me. That made me impatient. I saw the Mother in a vision. She spoke to me: "Do not be impatient, my child, he will be coming just now." I waited for some more time. But still you did not appear. That made me impatient all the more. I was on the point of weeping when the gracious Mother again consoled me. Soon a faint image of you rose up before me, and I began to take my food. What is this state?

SRI AUROBINDO: It is probably the growth of the need for some kind of contact of which the image is the vehicle.

Q: While offering my evening prayers, again I saw different images but they were vague and faint. How then to develop these images? Are they real?

SRI AUROBINDO: Nothing has to be done to develop them. They develop of themselves by the growing practice of seeing. What was faint becomes clear, what was incomplete becomes complete.

One cannot say in a general way that they are real or unreal.

Some are formations of the mind — some are images that come to the sight of themselves — some are images of real things that show themselves and, indirectly, to the sight — others are true pictures not merely images.

Q: Last night I saw you and LordKrishna in my dreams, but I forgot everything in the morning. When I woke up I was rather wondering whether I was sleeping or awake and whether I was meditating or seeing dreams! What was really that state?

SRI AUROBINDO: If I understand correctly what you write, it must be a state between the ordinary sleep and waking — but possibly a state of inner wakefulness, such as one gets when one goes inside in meditation.

Q: How to concentrate on the heart-centre?

SRI AUROBINDO: You can concentrate the consciousness any where in any centre. You have only to think of yourself as centrally there and try to fix and keep that. A strain or strong effort to do so is not necessary, a quiet and steady dwelling on the idea — after a time you will feel something there which you can recognise as consciousness steady and central and from there one can think, receive, originate action.

Most people associate consciousness with the brain or head because that is the centre for intellectual thought and mental vision, but consciousness is not limited to that kind of thought or vision, — it is everywhere in the system and there are several centres of it. *e.g.*, the centre for emotion is not in the brain but in the heart — the originating centre of vital desire is still lower down.

The two main places where one can centre the consciousness for Yoga are in the head and in the heart — the mind centre and the soul centre.

Q: On the night of the 11th I meditated for some time before going to bed. I soon felt as if there was a very bright sun. Its rays were passing through my chest and falling on Sri Aurobindo's picture-image present in my heart-centre. Due to the rays the picture-image began to shine so much that the reflection was dazzling my eyes! I began to ask myself what this was. Soon the idea came that I was having an experience. I got up, put on the light and, lest I should forget afterwards, wrote down a short account.

Now I want to ask you two questions. Was it really an experience? Would it have developed further had I not got up abruptly to note it down?

SRI AUROBINDO: The sun is the symbol of the concentrated light of Truth. The experience indicated that the light of Truth was entering into the heart centre and pressing for the change of your experiences which are still in the mind to the deeper spiritual experience which can be not merely a preparation but the firm foundation of your sadhana.

It is possible that something more might have happened — at any rate an experience should be allowed its full time whether to develop or have its full effect. It should not be interrupted except in case of necessity — or, of course, if it is not a good experience.

Q: Last evening I saw clear visions of Lord Krishna. This morning I saw Sri Aurobindo standing on a lotus. I talked and smiled to him. I also felt as if Lord Krishna was giving motion to the Sudarshan Chakra. What does it all indicate?

SRI AUROBINDO: These are the usual mental images. The chakra symbolises the action of Sri Krishna's force — the action of the Divine in you is already beginning to be clear and strong, but realisation of the Divine behind it is still faint.

16-9-1934

SRI AUROBINDO: To keep the consciousness awake you must set apart a certain time every day for concentration and remembering the Mother and keeping yourself in contact with us. What is gained is not lost by interruption, but it goes behind and may take time to come out again — so the thread should not be cut.

Your intuitions about the boy show that that faculty is awake in you; but you did not go because, as events proved, it was not necessary. The restlessness came from the vital; one should reject this reaction and act in perfect calm, keeping confidence in the Divine.

What you heard from inside is partly true. That is to say, there was no harm in taking advantage of any help you could get from the Maharaja; but there should be no eagerness; whatever offers itself should be taken as coming from the Mother. Eagerness disturbs the working of the forces and often creates obstacles.

Our blessings and protection are with you always.

Q: Sometimes I feel sleepy during meditation. Then the more I meditate the more strain I feel. Could you kindly show some means to avoid this sleep?

SRI AUROBINDO: I do not think the sleep can be avoided altogether. It will change by practice into a conscious inward condition in which you see and experience inner things.

Q: What is the best time for meditation?

SRI AUROBINDO: It depends on when one is most free.

Q: When in the outside world, I have to face certain worries: hospital duties, the ideas of my patients, my family troubles.

How to keep free from these anxieties?

SRI AUROBINDO: That is very difficult at the beginning. It is only by the concentration deepening until you get more and more absorbed inside in some inner experience that these things fall away.

Q: By this time you must have studied my nature well. Would you please give some directions to improve my inner consciousness?

SRI AUROBINDO: (1) Offer yourself more and more — all the consciousness, all that happens in it, all your work and action.

(2) If you have faults and weaknesses, hold them up before the Divine to be changed or abolished.

(3) Try to do what I told you, concentrate in the heart till you constantly feel the Presence there.

6-10-1934

SRI AUROBINDO: The weeping that rises in your offering of prayers is a psychic movement and a form of bhakti and aspiration welling up from within.

Keep a complete trust and work. You have a sufficient openness in you in your work for the Power to act; but a complete faith and courage are needed.

Our blessings are with you.

Q: During the Pranam ceremony the Mother meditates for a few minutes on what does she meditate?

SRI AUROBINDO: Whatever is needed for the sadhana the Mother concentrates to bring that down from the Divine.

Q: When the sadhak goes to her, looks at her and bows down to her, what does she say to him in silence?

SRI AUROBINDO: Whatever is needed for the individual sadhak and his progress.

Q: During that time, what is the significance of her pressing the occiput of the sadhak?

SRI AUROBINDO: It is usually to get rid of any resistance or obstacle that there may be in the mind — such as habits of thought, preconceived ideas, wrong notions, mental obscurity, inertia, etc.

6-5-1935

Q: Now I know the secret of the Pranam. When a sadhak bows down before the Mother, she sees in him the Mother-soul and prays to her to give him love, faith or anything else according to the meaning of the flower she gives to him. In this way a certain power is developed in the sadhak unconsciously. Am I right in this understanding?

SRI AUROBINDO: It is not quite like that. Mother puts the force into the sadhak and the power is felt by the sadhak sometimes consciously; but more often he receives it unconsciously. The sooner or later development of it depends on his condition and his response.

SRI AUROBINDO: I had no time to write as the time about the 24th. and after was very busy. I have received your letters and am glad to see that you are open to the Force and the work is proceeding well.

The experiences you have had indicate contact with the Mother Durga's force and reception of it. The red light round the heart is the light of that force.

I think it would be better not to put the photo in the book — let the book stand on its merit with the Force behind it.

The blessings of the Mother and mine are with you and yours.

14-8-1934

Q: This morning I was experiencing that Sri Aurobindo was doing **Yajna** *inside my body and the flames of the fire were very bright. What does it indicate?*

SRI AUROBINDO: It is an image of the Yoga, regarded as a sacrifice to the Divine. The fire is the fire of purification and Tapasya.

Q: Sri Aurobindo was taking me towards heaven in a **Viman** *(like an aeroplane) along a zig-zag way. I felt myself as if divided into two Agarwals — one with Sri Aurobindo and the other offering prayers below. First Sri Aurobindo took me to Lord Shiva and then to Lord Krishna. Both of us bowed at the Lord's feet. The Lord enquired about me and Sri Aurobindo said, "He is my Shishya (disciple)."*

SRI AUROBINDO: It is a mental formation trying to render some experience on the mental plane. The two Agarwals were two parts of your being. What was true experience was the ascent of the consciousness towards higher regions of consciousness.

Q: At the evening prayer time Mother Durga was standing and burning fire and it was all bright due to firelight. Then I saw a bright light coming from above and shining on my heart like a torch light. Then the heart became red and red light was inside. Its shape was like a red glass-box.

SRI AUROBINDO: The experiences indicate contact with the Mother Durga's force and reception of it. The red light round the heart is the light of that force.

Q: I was suffering from fever. In the night many fearful beings came before me though I was awake. I said to them, "I am under the protection of Sri Aurobindo. Sri Krishna's Sudershan Chakra will cut you in pieces." Then actually the Chakra appeared and was cutting them in pieces. At one time I saw a fire on a mountain.

Later on I saw Mother Durga telling me that I was under the protection of Sri Aurobindo. Then the Mother spoke to Sri Aurobindo, "I am much pleased with his bhakti, keep him under your special care." Then I saw Mother Mahalaxmi and the heart centre was shining and Sri Aurobindo was sitting there. What do these visions indicate?

SRI AUROBINDO: The illness you had and the depressing suggestions and fearful shapes came as an adverse attack, the other visions of the Powers of the Mother and the assurances you received were the answers that came through your psychic being calling the Divine. Whatever adverse things present themselves you must meet them with courage and they will disappear and the help come. Faith and courage are the true attitude to keep in life and work always and in the spiritual experience also. It is the fire of aspiration and the fire of faith and courage which you saw coming up from the mountain. The mountain is the symbol of embodied consciousness based upon the earth but rising up towards the Divine.

25-4-1935

Q: I was sitting in a cart and busy in my prayers to the Divine. Sri Aurobindo was taking the cart high up.

SRI AUROBINDO: The image of journeying always signifies a movement in life or a progress in sadhana.

31-7-1936

Q: A big light above my head and several other small lights were shining in the head and the vertebral column but the source of all of them was high above. Then I saw as if Sri Aurobindo was handling a bright flame in my heart. When I was absorbed in my meditation I was seeing some light around me. At one time a very bright light was descending and entering into my heart. Also I was feeling some sweet fragrance. What do these lights indicate?

SRI AUROBINDO: Lights or rays of light are always sign of the higher consciousness working in the being.

Q: I was going high up, at the top there was some light but not very distinct. The tears were flowing all the time. After the meditation I found the head heavy.

SRI AUROBINDO: Some part of consciousness must have gone up above.

Q: This morning during meditation I found myself sleeping. Then suddenly a fire-place with charcoal appeared and the red bright fire was peeping through the charcoal.

SRI AUROBINDO: It is a symbol of the condition in which there is the fire of aspiration below but there is *tamas* or dullness on the surface.

Q: While reading Bases of Yoga *I felt as if someone from inside was reading the book. Was it the psychic being?*

SRI AUROBINDO: No — the inner mental being.

14-8-1936

Q: Worldly thoughts were disturbing the meditation, so I imagined a 'Chakra' (round disk) moving fast around my head and preventing all thoughts entering into my head. Soon I found the mind quite silent and in deep meditation and experienced an intense light and the consciousness had a long upward journey.

What is the significance of this **Chakra** *?*

SRI AUROBINDO: A spiritual fire acting there.

Q: I was remembering the Divine Mother; soon a dark woman wearing a hat appeared before me and said, "I am Mother". I doubted and told her to go away. Then she disappeared.

SRI AUROBINDO: A power of darkness, I suppose such powers often try to pass themselves as the Mother or as the Divine or as one of the Godheads.

Q: I was seeing a silver swing on a lotus flower, on which the Divine Mother was sitting. A bright light appeared at the top of the silver and spread all around.

SRI AUROBINDO: A lotus flower indicates the open Consciousness.

17-8-1936

Q: Often I see in inner vision fire, lights, stars, light coming from the sun. Suddenly a bright sun appeared and the rays entered the head and I felt great heaviness. What do these lights indicate?

SRI AUROBINDO: Fire, lights, sun, moon are the usual symbols and seen by most in the sadhana. They indicate movement or action of inner forces — the sun means the inner truth.

THE END